CW01512714

NUTRIENT ESSENTIALS

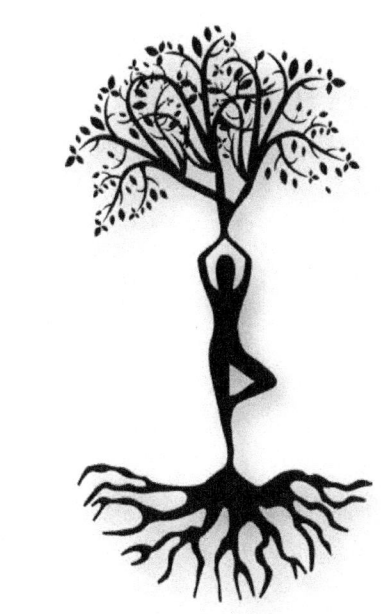

Judy Lickus

NUTRIENT ESSENTIALS

POLYUNSATURATED FATTY ACIDS ⎤
   OMEGA 6's + OMEGA 3's
    * OMEGA 6:3 RATIOS *   ⎬ FROM
   ALPHA LINOLENIC ACID   HIGH
   EPA and DHA ⎦ TO LOW

AMINO ACIDS ⎤
VITAMINS B ⎦   FOR OPTIMAL HEALTH

PROTEIN ⎤
FIBER
MONOUNSATURATED FATS ⎬ FROM HIGH TO LOW
SATURATED FATS ⎦

CALORIES ⎤
CARBOHYDRATE ⎬ FROM LOW TO HIGH
FATS ⎦

For the

PRACTICAL KITCHEN

By

JUDY LICKUS, B. Sc., LBSW

Published by JML Publishing
Corpus Christi, TX, USA 78404

Notice

The medical information in this book is provided as an educational resource only, and is not intended to be used or relied upon for any diagnosis or treatment purposes. This information should not be used as a substitute for professional diagnosis and treatment. The lifestyle interventions discussed in this book should not be used as a substitute for conventional medical treatment. None of the statements in this book have been evaluated by the Food and Drug Administration. It is sold with the understanding that the publisher and the author are not liable for the misconception or misuse of any information provided. Every effort has been made to make this book as complete and accurate as possible. The purpose of this book is to educate. This book is not intended as a substitute for any treatment prescribed by your doctor.

Mention of any particular company, organization, authority, or product manufacturer does not imply endorsement by the author or publisher, nor does mention of any specific company, organization, authority, or product manufacturer imply their endorsement of this book. Specific products and manufacturer information is shown to highlight variations among products, preparation, and manufacturers for the consumer food selection process.

Physical and internet addresses and directions cited in this book were accurate at the time this book went to press.

Any internet addresses or links are provided here solely for the sake of the reader. The author or the publisher are not affiliates of, nor do they receive any commissions from any of the resources mentioned in this book.

Copyright © 2019 by Judith Lickus, B. Sc., LBSW

All rights reserved. No part of this publication may be reproduced or transmitted in any form or by any means, graphic, electronic, or mechanical, including photocopying, recording, or by any other information storage and retrieval system, without the written permission of the publisher. Printed in the United States of America.

ISBN-9781795356411

Library of Congress Control Number: 2019906290

Published in Corpus Christi, Texas, USA by JML Publishing

TABLE OF CONTENTS

TABLE OF CHARTS

OVERVIEW

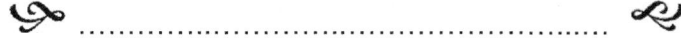

Using this book as your guide, you can easily design the
lifestyle changes that empower you to feel great and look
great when you eat health building foods that are
nutritious, delicious, and natural. Both your physical and mental
health will benefit with steady and reliable energy throughout your
days to reach your goals, live your dreams, and feel simply
awesome for life.

Designing your optimal nutrition is easy when you find all of the
data you need already mined for you and organized in unique ways
to assist you in locating just what you are looking for.

Inside the pages of this book you will find charts that unlock the
inner secrets of our foods. These resources can help you to
recapture your natural state of optimal health and well-being
naturally, without the use of potentially toxic pharmaceutical
products.

Ounces are the measurement used in all of the serving sizes for all
of the foods in all of the charts included in this book for the
practical kitchen. Metric guidance is also included throughout the
book. Plus there is an ounce to gram conversion chart for the
serving sizes used in this book included for added convenience.

Our bodies are so forgiving. They are powerful organisms capable
of healing themselves if given only half a chance. Imagine how
much greater we can be, when given greater than half a chance.

NUTRIENT ESSENTIALS

To enhance the functioning of our incredible bodies, we want to be sure to provide the essentials in the appropriate amounts. Our bodies actually need certain nutrients like essential fatty acids, essential amino acids, essential vitamins B, and minerals to live. These are the *nutrient essentials* that we must provide through our meal patterns.

We begin with the fatty acids (AKA fats), some of which are essential to our lives. We'll take a close look at each of the four basic types of fats we have to choose from: monounsaturated, polyunsaturated, saturated, and trans fats. Some of the oils and fats in our meal plans contain varying amounts of all four of these basic components. Then we will further study the micronutrients in some of the most important components. When we make our selections, it's a very personal situation, for many reasons that will become crystal clear as you read the first chapter.

We've learned through scientific research that our bodies need specific fats to do the jobs they are meant to do. They each have specific purposes in our well-being. It takes such a small amount of the right stuff to make a big difference in our health. It also takes such a small amount of the wrong stuff to deliver negative results in terms of our long-term health goals.

In this book, you'll find the richest food sources for each type of fat organized by the amount of the particular type of fat that they contain. For example, foods with the greatest amount of polyunsaturated fats are at the top of a polyunsaturated fats chart. Foods with the least amount of polyunsaturated fats are at the bottom of the chart. These charts are set up so you can compare the specific amounts of the important micronutrients that are in the different specific types of fats in our meal plans, for once and for all.

OVERVIEW

Special charts detail the *essential* polyunsaturated fatty acids (PUFA's) for you. You'll see detailed breakouts showing you the amounts of the different *types* of PUFA's such as linoleic, arachidonic, linolenic, EPA, and DHA in each of our polyunsaturated fats. You'll also learn the total amounts of both Omega 6's and Omega 3's that are in each type of fat. Furthermore, we will unlock the important Omega 6:3 ratios of each of our dietary polyunsaturated fats, listed in alphabetical order according to the name of the fats that contain them.

We'll further feature the most significant components of these fat types, noting the scientific research results pointing to the tremendous blessings of some, and the health destroying effects of others.

Next we'll look at protein, home of the *essential* amino acids. You'll see those that are essential, what our bodies do with them, and learn how to calculate your own personal recommended daily requirement for each of them for optimal health.

Some important protein sources, like nuts, seeds, and legumes (pulses) contain *phytic acid*, making that protein less available to many of us. You'll learn how you can easily increase the digestible protein, lower the carbohydrate content, and increase the amount of fiber in these types of vegetation.

We'll look at the *essential* vitamins B, which are just as important as the essential fatty acids and essential amino acids. You'll discover each one of these eight *nutrient essentials*, find out how they work together, and learn to recognize the symptoms of a deficiency in any one of them.

When we look at fruits, you'll learn about some of the most important antioxidant and anti-inflammatory properties in certain ones. You'll find out more about the work of bioflavonoids, vitamin C, and anthocyanins; why they are important, what they do for you, and some of the best fruits to focus on. You'll also find the fruits that serve you best if you have any of degree of concern regarding insulin resistance.

Throughout the book you'll find charts based on typical serving sizes, and see the amounts of the *macronutrients* they deliver. For instance, you'll see the calories, protein, carbohydrate, fiber, and fat in each of our different vegetables, nuts and seeds, legumes (pulses), grains, and fruits. Each of our groups of foods have a chart of their own, showing the foods in that group arranged in alphabetical order along with the amounts of macronutrients each of these foods contain listed right beside it. You are most likely already familiar with this type of chart.

For instance, let's say you have a *short term goal* of learning how much carbohydrate there is in a serving of cherries. The alphabetically organized *Fruit* chart lets your eye scan past the A and B listings until you get to those that begin with the letter C. You see that cherries have 14 grams of carbohydrate in a typical four and a quarter ounce serving. This meets your short term goal of learning the carbohydrate content of cherries. But what if you have a long term goal of eating less carbohydrate?

There is a special set of five uniquely organized charts designed especially for those who are looking for a different type of information because they have a certain *long term goal* in mind. These charts show you foods from a different *perspective*, and they have a special chapter of their own.

You may not be familiar with this type of chart. These charts organize and display foods from different perspectives.

For example, if your *long term goal* is to eat less *carbohydrate*, you can look at the *carbohydrate* chart for this point of view. In the carbohydrate chart, you can see how cherries compare with other foods in terms of the amount of carbohydrate they contain. As you look at this chart to locate cherries, you discover that strawberries (third entry from the top) have only 3 grams of carbohydrate for the same four and a quarter ounce serving as the cherries. You might very well decide to choose strawberries instead of cherries, and spare yourself those 11 extra grams of carbohydrate. And that is how these perspective charts can help you meet your specific long term goal of less carbohydrate.

You'll find a separate perspective chart for each of the basic components of our foods: calories, protein, carbohydrate, fiber, and fat. These charts list our foods from low to high (like calories and carbohydrate), or from high to low (like protein and fiber).

Finally, we will look at what it *really* takes to build and keep our strong bones. But it has little to do with dairy, a relatively poor source of absorbable calcium. Our bodies naturally stop producing *lactase*, the enzyme necessary to digest *lactose* after two to five years of age. That just so happens to coincide with nature's timeframe for the weaning of our young. Only humans consume the milk of another mammal after weaning from their mother's breast.

The fact is that over 60% of adults have a problem digesting *any* kind of dairy products. That means only 40% of adults are able to digest lactose. And as many as 75% of our African and Native Americans, and 90% of our Asian Americans have a condition known as "lactose intolerance."

What happens is that the undigested milk sugars end up in our colons where they begin ferment, creating significant issues. To assist the normally lactose intolerant individual, in this book you will find a chart of lactose containing foods. And yet another chart lists some popular creative names used by the food industry to

5

disguise the presence of lactose in our foods, to help you avoid them.

For the normally lactose sensitive individual, we'll be looking at natural ways to assure our calcium absorption for our strong bones.

In our Strong Bones Recipes, you'll even learn about some minerals you will want to include – and others you will want to avoid in your meal plans and preparations. You'll also read about some commonly used toxic products, and see a list of ways to help you replace them.

For women, we'll be taking a look at menopause. You'll learn about some of the different hormone replacement options that are available to support bone strength (and more) to assure strong and satisfactory aging. Plus a simple test you can get before menopause begins in order to avoid the confusion, depression, and many of the other unnecessary symptoms of this time of life.

We finish our look at strong bones with some simple exercises that will help anyone develop better balance and bone strength. These exercises are so easy that even a child can do them, and they are so much fun to do that they will surely want to. But in spite of the ease, these simple exercises strengthen your bones and increase your balance naturally. Regardless of age or physical condition, anyone can enhance the development of their strong bones for a long, healthy active life.

No two bodies are alike. We are each unique in all of the world. Each of us has slightly different requirements to meet as we fulfill our needs of the *nutrient essentials*. And since food becomes one with our bodies, it is important to understand the nature of the foods we eat to nourish our naturally awesome bodies and simply live our dreams.

FATTY ACIDS

MY Plate guidelines recommend 5 – 7 teaspoons (2 tablespoons, or about 28 g.) of oil each day, or 10% of our calories be from fats. Oils are not given a food group of their own on the plate. Instead, it is expected that we will consume them as part of our salad dressings, cooking oils, and in the nuts and fish we eat. Fatty acids really do deserve a whole lot more respect than that. But what exactly are these fats, and how do we select those that best serve our health?

There are four basic types of dietary fatty acids: Saturated, monounsaturated, polyunsaturated, and trans fats. Some of the oils and fats in our meal plans contain varying amounts of all four of these basic components. And when we make our selections, it's absolutely not a "one size fits all" situation, either, for many reasons that will become crystal clear in this chapter.

For over half a century we were told that all fats, especially saturated fats, were the cause of coronary artery disease. We were told to cut back on them or avoid them entirely.

It all started with a tug of war between Ancel Keys, an American physiologist (Author of the Seven Countries Study in 1958), and the British physiologist John Yudkin (Author of Pure White and Deadly in 1972, recently resurrected by Robert Lustig with a new introduction[1] and much too late to avoid the fat-removal spree supported by Keys.) Keys was instrumental in promoting the big fat lie sponsored by the sugar industry.

Manufacturers took the fats from many of our foods. Added sugar, hydrogenated fats, and refined carbohydrates replaced fats to make up for the loss of energy (calories) the naturally occurring fats provided. This scenario played out over the course of over fifty years. It also handily orchestrated many of our current epidemics. Non-communicable disease epidemics like obesity, heart disease, insulin resistance, type 2 diabetes, many types of cancer, and other disorders present in our society today can thank the sugar industries lobbying efforts for their popularity today.

Finally, we are beginning to look at some of the details of our fats and learn that they might be just the nutrient we need more of. And since the fat-removal necessity spell has now been broken, we will look at some recent research, as well as some of the older study results focusing on very specific fatty acids to help us define our own individualized program of a new way to better health.

For some dietary fats, research is pretty skimpy in terms of human consumption, likely because we had, for so long, abandoned fats all we possibly could. In spite of the results of the great abandonment of fats, many fats consistently demonstrate their health blessing properties, regardless of earlier errant public health recommendations that grew out of the efforts of Ancel Keys and the sugar industry.

Even our first Food Pyramid, published by the USDA in the early 1980's recommended we eat some eight to eleven servings of carbohydrate a day. We had silos full of grains to supply demand, and grains were very inexpensive. Carbohydrates formed the very base of that first pyramid, depicted by loaves of breads, piles of pasta and bowls of rice. After over a quarter century run, the pyramid was replaced by the plate that we use today. But something is missing from the picture. There is no image to represent fats as a recommended portion, and our health building meal plans must include certain essential fatty acids.

In June, 2012, Thomas Seyfried published his work, *Cancer as a Metabolic Disease*[2], dealing with brain cancer, an organ with little circulation. His book changed everything. How could we not begin to wonder what other diseases are sparked by errant metabolic processes caused by fatless meal plans?

As scientific researchers began to dust off and review some of the older studies with new eyes, they discovered that many suspect fats are really good for us. In some cases, research databases allow scientists to view the dietary patterns of large groups of people over long periods of time and compare long-term health outcomes. Scientists used dietary questionnaires to keep track of the types of foods these subjects consumed and see their health consequences after several decades. These health questionnaires allow researchers to look back and notice trends in food choices to see how they affect long term public health. We'll be looking at some of their findings later in this chapter.

But hold on a minute. Let's go back a step. Just because we need some fatty acids for our health, doesn't mean we need to consume large amounts of them. The fact is that most of us don't need a lot of fats compared to the amount, in terms of volume, of other foods on our plate, like protein, calcium, vegetables, fruits, and whole grains. And fats have over twice as many calories (9) as protein or carbohydrate (4 each).

For perspective, an entire apple (about 4 ¼ oz. or 120 g.) contains as much energy (calories) as just a mere Tbsp. (.5 oz. or 14 g.) of most fats. But some of these fats so very important to our health that we call them "essential fatty acids." They are essential because we can't live without them. So it's important to include them in our meal plans.

Just 1 to 2 tablespoons a day may do the job quite well for most of us. That's because the right fats are so powerful that just a small amount is all that we really need for our optimum health. The reverse is also true. It takes just a small amount of the wrong fats to damage our health, as well. So we're going to put them in the spotlight to get a closer look and create a better understanding.

In the first chart, Figure 1, we'll warm up to the different fatty acid foods to see just what some of our options are. We'll see exactly how many calories and how much total fat there really is in each of 51 popular food sources of fatty acids. They are all measured in 1 tablespoon (.5 oz. or about 14 g.) serving sizes.

The foods listed in the first column are the oils obtained from those listed foods. In other words, the entry "Almond" is for Almond oil, which is the oil that is extracted from almonds, etc. This is true for all of the fatty acids in all of the fatty acid charts in this book. All of the serving sizes are 1 tablespoon, .5 oz., or 14 g.

The second column of the first fatty acid chart, below, presents the number of calories that are in that size serving. And the third column shows you the amount of total fat in that serving of that food, regardless of the type of fat (saturated, monounsaturated, polyunsaturated, or trans) that it is. We'll get to that in a bit.

{*Note: The information in all of the charts that is given for each type of animal fat is just for the pure fat portion of that animal. It does not include muscle meats or any portion thereof, just the fat, pure and simple, so we can compare one fat to another fat. Period.}
~ *End of note.

FATTY ACIDS

The information in this chart is organized alphabetically by the name of each food:

Figure 1: FATTY ACIDS CALORIES + FAT

Oils, AKA Fatty Acids 1 Tbsp./.5 Oz./ ≈14 g.	Cal	Fat g.
Algae	120	14
Almond	120	13.60
Apricot kernel	120	13.60
Avocado	124	14
Babassu	120	13.60
Bacon grease	116	12.84
Beef fat	115	12.80
Butter	102	11.52
Butter, clarified	112	12.50
Canola	130	15
Canola for commercial deep frying	120	13.60
Chicken fat	115	12.77
Cocoa butter	120	13.60
Coconut, virgin	120	14.00
Coconut, refined	130	14.00
Corn	120	13.50
Cottonseed	120	13.60
Extra Virgin Olive	120	14
Fish, cod liver	123	13.60
Fish, herring	123	13.60
Fish, menhaden	123	13.60
Fish, salmon	123	13.60
Fish, sardine	123	13.60
Flax seed	130	14
Goose fat	115	12.77
Grape Seed	140	15
Hazelnut	120	13.60
Hemp, cold pressed	124	14

Oils, AKA Fatty Acids 1 Tbsp./.5 Oz./ ≈14 g.	Cal	Fat g.
Lamb fat	92	9.76
Lard	115	12.80
Mustard	124	14
Oat	120	13.60
Olive	120	13.50
Palm	120	13.60
Palm kernel	117	13.60
Peanut	130	14
Poppyseed	120	13.60
Pork fat	89	9.28
Rice bran	120	13.60
Safflower	120	14
Salmon oil	123	13.60
Sheanut	120	13.60
Soybean	120	14
Soybean lecithin	104	13.60
Sunflower	124	14
Teaseed	120	13.60
Tomato seed	120	13.60
Turkey fat	115	12.77
Veal fat	72	7.37
Walnut	120	13.60
Wheat Germ	120	13.60

[3,4]

Now that we have an idea of just how many calories and grams of fat there are in these foods, we can get started looking at more specifics. We'll cover each of these different fatty acid food sources foods in detail throughout this chapter. Plus you might find some new ideas that are useful in increasing the most healthful in your diet.

It's a very personal and specific situation. As a matter of fact, according to the latest research, published by the journal *Nutrients* in July, 2018, "supplementation with different fatty acid compositions resulted in specific responses."[5] So it is important to get the right fats for the sake of your own personal highest health over a lifetime. That's why you will find detailed break out charts showing you the amounts of the different components of the individual fatty acids presented in this book.

And we will start with the simplest, the monounsaturated fatty acids.

MONOUNSATURATED FATS

Monounsaturated fats became popular in the 1960's when scientists discovered that people with a high intake of olive oil had reduced rates of heart disease. This sparked the birth of the popular Mediterranean diet. These fats are liquid at room temperature. They are solid or semi-solid when refrigerated.

And it is no wonder that monounsaturated fats are promoted as healthy. Going back to a 2011 study published by *Lipids,* authors report "Consumption of dietary MUFA [MonoUnsaturated Fatty Acids] promotes healthy blood lipid profiles, mediates blood pressure, improves insulin sensitivity and regulates glucose levels."[6]

In terms of cancer, the journal *Medicine* published a study in 2016 on the dietary fat intake of 524,583 subjects gathered from other studies. The authors of this study found that "Results from the cohort studies suggested higher monounsaturated fatty acid intake was significantly associated with lower endometrial cancer risk."[7]

Finally, in a study published in January, 2018, by the journal *Oxidative Medicine and Cellular Longevity*, the authors write, "The best dietary advice for the prevention and management of obesity and other metabolic disorders includes replacing refined carbohydrates with whole grains, increasing fruits and vegetables, substituting total and saturated fat with MUFAs [monounsaturated fatty acids]."[8]

Good sources of monounsaturated fats are almonds, avocados, cashews, cold pressed extra virgin olive oil, olives, and peanuts. Coconut oil and palm kernel oil are very poor sources.

A Better Butter recipe for the practical kitchen: Combining equal amounts of butter and extra virgin olive oil makes a delicious easy-to-spread topping. Just let your butter warm to room temperature until it becomes softened and combine in a blender with an equal amount of olive oil. Pour your spread into a container and store in the refrigerator. It will act much like margarine. Use as a spread, and for cooking over low heat. You can use another mild flavored monounsaturated oil to mix with your butter, if you prefer.

This is a simple way to include more monounsaturated fat in the diets of those who are tolerant of dairy. Having a container already mixed makes it easy and convenient to increase these monounsaturated fats in our diets. Every serving used in cooking or dressing provides an equal amount of monounsaturated as well as saturated fat.

Now we will organize our fatty acid foods by the amount of monounsaturated fats they contain. All serving sizes are for .5 oz., 1 Tablespoon, or 14 g.

For all food sources in our charts, it is the oil from that particular food, or the fat portion of the animal that is being charted. This is the first time in this book that we will use a unique way to display our fatty acids. Foods with the greatest amount of monounsaturated fatty acids are shown at the top of the chart. The foods with the least amount of monounsaturated fats are shown at the bottom of the chart:

FATTY ACIDS

Figure 2: MONOUNSATURATED FATS

Oils, AKA Fatty Acids 1 Tbsp./.5 Oz/ ≈14 g	Monounsaturated g
Algae	13
Sunflower	11.70
Safflower	11
Hazelnut	10.61
Extra Virgin Olive	10
Olive	9.9
Avocado	9.88
Canola for commercial deep frying	9.67
Almond	9.50
Canola	8.86
Mustard	8.29
Apricot kernel	8.16
Fish, herring	7.69
Goose fat	7.26
Peanut	7
Teaseed	7
Fish, cod liver	6.35
Sheanut	5.98
Bacon grease	5.79
Lard	5.77
Chicken fat	5.72
Turkey fat	5.49
Rice bran	5.35
Palm	5.03
Oat	4.78
Fish, sardine	4.60
Cocoa butter	4.47
Corn	4
Beef fat	3.96
Pork fat	3.96
Fish, salmon	3.95
Lamb fat	3.95
Salmon oil	3.95
Fish, menhaden	3.63
Butter	3.33
Walnut	3.18

Oils, AKA Fatty Acids 1 Tbsp./.5 Oz/ ≈14 g	Monounsaturated g
Tomato seed	3.10
Soybean	3
Veal fat	2.94
Poppyseed	2.68
Cottonseed	2.42
Wheat Germ	2.05
Flax seed	2
Hemp, cold pressed	1.99
Palm kernel	1.55
Babassu	1.51
Soybean lecithin	1.5
Coconut, virgin	1
Coconut, refined	1

[9, 10]

Before we continue, there is a word of caution. When cooking with any oil, it is important to use low heat. Low heat allows you to retain and not destroy any polyunsaturated fats an oil may contain. Polyunsaturated fats are famously known for their health benefits. We'll be looking a lot closer at these polyunsaturated fats next, after we talk about the ways we use fats and oils in our kitchens.

When an oil gets close to its' smoke point[11] it begins to break down – causing it to oxidize and produce free radicals, much as many oils do when subjected to the refining process.

These free radicals are toxins that can damage our healthy cells. This is a form of oxidative stress, and a good reason to assure that we get enough antioxidants. Antioxidants are front line defenders and may slow, stop, or even prevent aging, cancer, allergies, and other diseases.

The breaking down process caused by heating fats may convert some of the delicate polyunsaturated fatty acids into trans fats. This is a common side effect of the deep frying operations used in commercial kitchens. We will look more closely at this later.

FATTY ACIDS

There are nearly as many different "smoke points" as there are oils. In some cases, refined oils may have higher smoke points than unrefined, natural oils. In other cases, the reverse may be true. But refined oils have already been irreversibly damaged during the refining process. This little chart highlights some of the approximate smoke points you may well like to keep in mind when cooking with these fats:

Figure 3: SMOKE POINTS OF COOKING OILS

Oil	Unrefined	Refined
Almond	430	
Avocado	480	520
Butter	302	
Canola	225	400
Coconut	350	450
Corn	352	446
Extra Virgin Olive	320	390-470
Grapeseed	421	
Lard	374	
Safflower	225	510
Sunflower	225	486-489

12

ESSENTIAL FATTY ACIDS: POLYUNSATURATED FATS

Polyunsaturated fats are those *essential* fatty acids we hear so much about. They are called essential fatty acids because they are indispensable -- our bodies can't make them, so we need to get them from our foods.

How can you tell if you are not getting enough of these essentials? One easily recognized clue according to the resource *Dietary reference intakes for energy, carbohydrate, fiber, fat, fatty acids, cholesterol, protein, and amino acids (macronutrients)* published by our Institute of Medicine, Food and Nutrition Board, "A deficiency of essential fatty acids—either omega-3s or omega-6s—can cause rough, scaly skin and dermatitis"[13]

Healthy, radiant skin is an obvious reason to assure an adequate supply of polyunsaturated fatty acids, but it turns out that there is so much more we can be grateful for when we keep up with our polyunsaturated fatty acid intake. What else do we need polyunsaturated fatty acids for?

In a 2015 study published by the International *Journal of Molecular Science*, scientists state, "Recent studies have clearly shown the important impact of polyunsaturated fatty acids (PUFAs) on human health in the prevention of, particularly, cardiovascular disease (CVD), coronary heart disease and cancer; further, inflammatory, thrombotic and autoimmune disease; hypertension; diabetes type two, renal diseases; and rheumatoid arthritis, ulcerative colitis, and Crohn's disease."[14]

It is the polyunsaturated fatty acids that are the all-stars. But what are these polyunsaturated fats, and how can we be sure to get the right amount of them? It turns out that there are a couple different groups of them. And since they are so important, we're going to drill down a lot closer to unlock the secrets of these most healthful fats, these polyunsaturated fatty acids.

A sequence of charts will break out the specifics. Here's what you will see: In Figure 5, you'll see a breakout of 44 foods that contain delicate polyunsaturated fatty acids (PUFAs). The first chart shows just how much polyunsaturated fats these fats contain. You'll see the foods with the highest amount of polyunsaturated fats right at the top of the chart. Foods with the least amount of polyunsaturated fats are at the bottom of the chart.

Figure 6 shows the Omega 6's, the total amounts of linoleic and arachidonic (two Omega 6's) fatty acids, and the total amount of Omega 6's in each particular dietary source. Foods with the highest levels of Omega 6 polyunsaturated fats are at the top of this chart. Foods with the least amount of Omega 6 polyunsaturated fatty acids are at the bottom of the chart.

Figure 7 is a chart for one of the Omega 3's, Alpha Linolenic Acid (ALA). The foods with the greatest amount of ALA are at the top of the chart. Those with the least amount of ALA are at the bottom of the chart.

Figure 8 shows you a breakout into the amounts of the specific components of the Omega 3's: Alpha Linolenic Acid (ALA), eicosapentaeoic acid (EPA), and docosahexaenoic acid (DHA), and the total Omega 3's in each particular source. Foods with the highest level of total Omega 3's are at the top of this chart. Foods with the least amount of total Omega 3's are at the bottom of the chart.

Figure 9 details EPA and DHA, both being Omega 3 polyunsaturated fatty acids.

The final stop in our tour of polyunsaturated fatty acids is Figure 10. In figure 10, you will see the Omega 6:3 Ratio for each of the fats in our food sources.

Then we'll cover saturated fats and trans fats to complete a thorough review of the fatty acids in our lives. You'll find research results along the way showing the important roles of many factors involved in our fat intake, and consider the contributions they make to our lifelong health, well-being, and happiness.

You may be wondering why it is important to get into this much detail. Couldn't we just look at some of the basics to pick a winner? Maybe not in today's world where there are so many celebrities promoting fad diets for "miracle" cures that may never arrive. Are they promoting the products they have for sale, or offering real scientific information upon which individuals can make decisions?

Our bodies are so forgiving. They are powerful organisms capable of healing themselves when given only half a chance. Imagine how much better we can be, when given a greater than half a chance.

Science has proven that our bodies need specific lipids (fats) to do the jobs they are meant to do. They each have specific purposes in our well-being. It takes such a small amount of the right stuff to make a big difference in our health. It also takes such a small amount of the wrong stuff to deliver negative results in terms of our long-term health goals.

Now we'll begin our focus on some of the greatest healers we can offer to our bodies, the polyunsaturated fats. The chart below organizes our fatty acid food sources by the amount of polyunsaturated fats they contain. The foods with the highest amount of polyunsaturated fatty acids are at the top of the chart. The foods with the least amount of polyunsaturated fatty acids are at the bottom of the chart. For all food sources in our charts, it is the oil from that particular food, or the fat portion of the animal that is being charted. All of the data here is given for a 1 Tbsp. serving size, or one half ounce (or about 14 g.).

Figure 4: ESSENTAIL POLYUNSATURATED FATS

Oils, AKA Fatty Acids 1 Tbsp. =.5 Oz/ ≈14 g	Polyunsaturated g.
Hemp, cold pressed	11
Flax seed	10
Grape Seed	10
Soybean	9
Walnut	8.61
Poppyseed	8.49
Wheat Germ	8.39
Corn	7.50
Tomato seed	7.22
Cottonseed	7.06
Soybean lecithin	6.2
Oat	5.56
Fish, salmon	5.48
Salmon oil	5.48
Peanut	5
Rice bran	4.76
Fish, menhaden	4.65
Fish, sardine	4.33
Apricot kernel	3.99
Canola	3.94
Teaseed	3.13
Fish, cod liver	3.07
Turkey fat	2.98
Mustard	2.97
Chicken fat	2.68
Almond	2.37
Fish, herring	2.12
Safflower	1.99
Canola for commercial deep frying	1.91
Avocado	1.88

Oils, AKA Fatty Acids 1 Tbsp. =.5 Oz/ ≈14 g	Polyunsaturated g.
Extra Virgin Olive	1.5
Bacon grease	1.44
Lard	1.43
Goose fat	1.41
Olive	1.4
Hazelnut	1.39
Palm	1.27
Pork fat	1.09
Sheanut	.71
Algae	.500
Butter, clarified	0.50
Sunflower	.50
Butter	.43
Cocoa butter	.41
Beef fat	0.40
Lamb fat	0.40
Coconut, virgin	.231
Coconut, refined	.231
Veal fat	0.23
Babassu	0.22
Palm kernel	0.22

15, 16

Now that we can see how much polyunsaturated fat is in these fats, we can break out the specific *types* of polyunsaturated fatty acids (PUFA's) we are looking at in each of these fats. Please note that the amounts of overall PUFA's in each are measured in grams, as you can see in the above chart. The amounts of the different types of PUFA's we will be looking at are measured in milligrams.

There are two main types of polyunsaturated fatty acids we will be looking at here. They are the Omega 6 and Omega 3 fatty acids. Your body uses them to build things like nerve coverings and cell membranes. They are also used for blood clotting, muscle movements, and inflammation or … anti-inflammation.

FATTY ACIDS

These polyunsaturated fats are the natural ingredients that can reduce blood pressure, LDL cholesterol (the bad kind) levels and lower our triglyceride levels. They are also known for their impact on brain function and cognitive health. These nutritional treasures are complex because they are composed of many parts. In order to establish an understanding of the whole, we must first create understanding of the various parts.

That's because there is a trick to these essential fatty acids. The trick is that we need them in the correct *balance* in order to protect our hearts, pancreas, joints, skin, and our precious moods. So to do justice to the allocation of which polyunsaturated fatty acids we want to include in our diets, we have to break out some of the specifics. And we'll start with Omega 6 polyunsaturated fats.

OMEGA 6 FATTY ACIDS

Unfortunately, in terms of meeting the correct balance, we get way too many Omega 6's from the corn and vegetable oils used in so many of our commercially prepared foods. This is particularly so whenever we consume many of the processed foods so easily available today. And it's not just "fast foods," that we are singling out here, it also includes foods prepared by restaurants and delicatessens. The fact is that we don't know what types of fats or oils are used in the preparation of our foods when we dine at these places. And we can't live on plain salads alone.

While Omega 6 fatty acids may take away the rash on our skin, Omega 6's can also cause our bodies to retain water, raise our blood pressure, and may even lead to blood clots that can cause heart attacks and strokes.

That's because Omega 6's can cause inflammation, the root of many of our non-communicable diseases like heart disease, cancer, obesity, and T2D. So maybe we'd like to avoid fats that are high in

Omega 6 fatty acids. These include corn, cottonseed, safflower, soybean, and regular "vegetable oil," (whatever that *really* is). This is particularly true if we are experiencing any type of inflammation.

Biomed Pharmacotherapy published an article in 2002 titled "The importance of the ratio of omega-6/omega-3 essential fatty acids." In this article, Artemis Simopoulos explains how we evolved from a natural Omega 6:3 ratio of 1:1. The ideal ratio, then, is our natural ratio of 1:1. Yet today most of us have a ratio of over 15:1. That means for every fifteen tablespoons of Omega 6 we consume, we consume only one tablespoon of Omega 3 fatty acids.

Scientists have learned that our current 15:1 ratio is really good -- to "promote the pathogenesis of many diseases, including cardiovascular disease, cancer, and inflammatory and autoimmune diseases."[17] And further, "a lower ratio of omega-6/omega-3 fatty acids is more desirable in reducing the risk of many of the chronic diseases of high prevalence in Western societies, as well as in the developing countries, that are being exported to the rest of the world."[18]

So we want to hunt down just how much of Omega 6 fatty acids we are consuming, and find out exactly where they are found among our polyunsaturated fatty acids.

The next chart gives us a break out of the main components of Omega 6 polyunsaturated fatty acids. In this chart, we can see the amount of Linoleic Acid (LA) and arachidonic, as well as the total amount of Omega 6's in the food sources listed in the left hand column. The amounts of each type of Omega 6 are listed in milligrams (mg.). Then the Total amount of Omega 6's in each of these sources is listed in the right hand column. The foods are arranged by those with the highest amount of total Omega 6 fatty acids at the top of the chart. Hopefully this arrangement may help you avoid them. Foods with the least amount of total Omega 6's are at the bottom of the chart. Keep in mind that it is the oil from the listed food or the fat portion only from an animal source. All of the serving sizes are 1 tablespoon, ½ oz. or about 14 g.:

Figure 5: TOTAL OMEGA 6 FATTY ACIDS

FATTY ACID .5 oz. = 1 Tbsp.= ≈14 g.	LINOLEIC mg.	ARACHID ONIC mg.	TOTAL OMEGA 6 mg.
Grape Seed	9466	0	9466
Poppyseed	8486	0	8486
Corn			7224
Walnut	7194	0	7194
Cottonseed	7004	14	7018
Tomato seed	6909	0	6909
Sesame	5617	0	5617
Soybean lecithin	5465	0	5465
Sunflower	5413	0	5413
Oat	5315	0	5315
Rice bran	4542	0	4542
Peanut	4320	0	4320
Apricot kernel	3985	0	3985
Teaseed	3019	0	3019
Chicken fat	2500	381	2881
Turkey fat	2714	38	2752
Canola	2661	0	2661
Wheat Germ	2466	0	2466
Almond	2370	0	2370
Mustard	2146	0	2146
Flax seed	1900	0	1900
Avocado	1754	0	1754
Safflower	1730	0	1730
Canola for commercial deep frying	1706	0	1706
Pork fat	1670	26	1696
Hazelnut	1374	0	1374
Olive	1318	0	1318
Bacon grease	1310	0	1310

FATTY ACID .5 oz. = 1 Tbsp.= ≈14 g.	LINOLEIC mg.	ARACHID ONIC mg.	TOTAL OMEGA 6 mg.
Lard	1306	0	1306
Goose fat	1254	0	1254
Sheanut	666	0	666
Fish, sardine	274	239	513
Fish, menhaden	293	159	452
Beef fat	397	0	397
Cocoa butter	381	0	381
Fish, salmon	210	92	302
Lamb fat	234	37	271
Butter	260	0	260
Fish, cod liver	127	127	254
Coconut	229	0	229
Babassu	220	0	220
Palm kernel	218	0	218
Fish, herring	156	39	195
Veal fat	165	4	169

[19, 20, 21]

Now that we have a general idea of how much total Omega 6 might be in our diet, we're going to look at one of the Omega 3 fatty acids. After that we will create a total of all Omega 3 fatty acids, just like we did for the Omega 6's.

OMEGA 3 FATTY ACIDS

The first Omega 3 fatty acid we want to look at is Alpha Linolenic Acid. It deserves special recognition because of its measurable effects on cardiovascular biomarkers, especially high LDL levels, judged to be a warning for stroke and heart disease.

Consider this 2015 study published by the journal *Nutrition*. Researchers gave two groups of subjects .35 oz., (about one third of an ounce, or about 10 g.) of two different kinds of oil each day. The researchers aimed to check on the biological effect of the Omega 3 polyunsaturated fat, Alpha Linolenic Acid (ALA) on cardiovascular risk factors. To conduct their experiment, one group of subjects had flaxseed oil (containing 5.45 g. or 5450 mg. of ALA), and the other group had corn oil (containing 0.09 g. or 90 mg. of ALA). Each group had their serving of oil with dinner each day. The length of the study was four months. They researchers concluded, "FO [flaxseed oil], which is a rich source of ALA and EPA, leads to dramatically lower sd-LDL cholesterol concentrations."[22] – The corn oil, according to the researchers, had no effect.

What is most powerful about this study is that it shows that ALA delivered positive cardiovascular results. This is particularly important because seafood may not always available. Previous studies delivered conflicting analysis on whether the body could actually metabolize sufficient EPA and DHA from the ALA for positive cardiovascular protective effects. We'll look closer at EPA and DHA later.

In terms of public health, like yours and mine, we can see from the above study that the cardio protective effect provided by a rich source of alpha linolenic acid (ALA) delivers a most positive result in a relatively short period of time.

Since the polyunsaturated Omega 3 fat, Alpha Linolenic Acid (ALA) can have such a dramatic effect in lowering LDL cholesterol (the bad kind), it warrants our special recognition and coverage.

So here comes a chart speaking directly to the wonderful results in the above study. Only fatty acid food sources that contain ALA are included in this chart. There are 37 of them, down 14 from the 51 fats we looked at in Figure 1 earlier. The amount of ALA in these fats is measured in milligrams (mg.) Foods with the greatest amount of ALA are at the top of the chart. Foods with the least amount of ALA are at the bottom of the chart. The serving size is 1 tablespoon, .5 oz., or about 14 g.:

27

NUTRIENT ESSENTIALS

Figure 6: ALPHA LINOLENIC ACID

FATTY ACID .5 oz. = 1 Tbsp.= ≈14 g.	LINOLENIC (ALA) mg.
Flax seed	7640
Walnut	1414
Canola	1279
Mustard	826
Soybean lecithin	698
Tomato seed	313
Wheat Germ	310
Oat	243
Rice bran	218
Fish, menhaden	203
Canola for commercial deep frying	200
Fish, sardine	180
Turkey fat	179
Butter	168
Fish, salmon	144
Avocado	130
Chicken fat	130
Bacon grease	129
Lard	128
Fish, cod liver	127
Lamb fat	113
Fish, herring	104
Olive	103
Teaseed	95
Pork fat	83
Beef fat	77
Goose fat	64
Veal fat	46
Sesame	41
Sheanut	41
Cottonseed	27
Sunflower	27
Corn	20
Cocoa butter	14
Grape Seed	14
Safflower	13

FATTY ACID .5 oz. = 1 Tbsp.= ≈14 g.	LINOLENIC (ALA) mg.
Coconut	3

[23], [24], [25]

As you can see in the above chart, flax seed, walnut, and canola are the best sources of alpha-linolenic acid (ALA). And flax seed, at the top of the chart, delivers over *five times* more ALA than the second in line, walnut.

Other sources of ALA include kale, Brussels sprouts, cauliflower, kohlrabi, parsley, and carrots.

High cholesterol levels affect about 29 million Americans today. And high LDL cholesterol (the bad kind) concentration is thought to be a major warning signal for coronary heart disease, potentially leading to heart attack and stroke. And if adding a bit of flax seed to our daily diets is all it takes to lower our cholesterol levels, is there really any reason to settle for using statin prescription medications (along with their side effects) to give us a lower cholesterol reading?

And such a small amount is all it takes. Flax seed, purchased from a health food type store, where it is stored in the refrigerator or freezer, is easily incorporated into a smoothie. You can prepare your smoothie the night before, allowing the flax seed to soak in the liquid overnight. Strive for organic, pure & unrefined flax seed. It is best consumed fresh, and can be added as a crunchy topping to a nice fresh salad. You can also grind it in a coffee grinder, Nutribullet, or Ninja, before adding it to your smoothie or just before using it. It can be used for cooking, creating a crunchy coating for chicken or fish. But it is best to consume flax seed fresh for the greatest benefit.

The ratio of omega 6:3 in the oil of flax seed is about 1:7. That means for every one drop of Omega 6 there are seven drops of

Omega 3 fatty acids. But we can do even more than that, especially where our hearts are concerned. And we will cover that when we look at the Omega 6 to Omega 3 ratio, coming up soon.

While we consider how we will keep the oils in our lives in balance, it is important to note that the Omega 6's and Omega 3's compete with each other for use in our bodies. So if we consume a lot of Omega 6's then the Omega 3's we do get may hardly stand a chance. And another reason why that balance is so important.

It is the Omega 3's that our bodies really need to build our health. So now we'll break out those wonderful health building Omega 3's even further. We will also focus on those that have the most scientific evidence demonstrating their place of honor in our meal plans.

There are three basic types of Omega 3 fatty acids that we will be looking at in this next chart: Alpha Linolenic acid (ALA), eicosapentaenoic acid (EPA), and docosahexaenoic acid (DHA), and the total Omega 3's in each food source.

All of the data here is given for a 1 Tbsp. serving size, or .50 oz. or 14 g. The components of each type of these three Omega 3 polyunsaturated fatty acids are listed in milligrams (mg.). Our food sources are listed here in the order of the most to the least amount of total Omega 3's. Those with the greatest amount of Total Omega 3's are at the top of the chart. Those with the least amount of Total Omega 3's are at the bottom of the chart:

Figure 7: OMEGA 3 FATTY ACIDS

FATTY ACID .5 oz. = 1 Tbsp.= ≈14 g.	ALPHA LINOLE NIC (ALA) mg.	EPA mg.	DHA mg.	TOTAL OMEGA 3 mg.
Flax seed	7640	0	0	7640

FATTY ACIDS

FATTY ACID .5 oz. = 1 Tbsp.= ≈14 g.	ALPHA LINOLE NIC (ALA) mg.	EPA mg.	DHA mg.	TOTAL OMEGA 3 mg.
Fish, salmon	144	1771	2480	4395
Fish, menhaden	203	1791	1164	3158
Fish, sardine	180	1379	1449	3008
Fish, herring	104	853	572	1529
Walnut	1414	0	0	1414
Canola	1279	0	0	1279
Fish, cod liver	127	938	127	1192
Mustard	826	0	0	826
Soybean lecithin	698	0	0	698
Tomato seed	313	0	0	313
Wheat Germ	310	0	0	310
Oat	243	0	0	243
Rice bran	218	0	0	218
Canola for commercial deep frying	200	0	0	200
Turkey fat	179	0	0	179
Butter	168	0	0	168
Corn				157
Avocado	130	0	0	130
Chicken fat	130	0	0	130
Bacon grease	129	0	0	129
Lard	128	0	0	128
Lamb fat	113	0	0	113
Olive	103	0	0	103
Teaseed	95	0	0	95
Pork fat	83	0	7	90
Beef fat	77	0	0	77
Goose fat	64	0	0	64
Veal fat.	46	2	10	58
Sheanut	41	0	0	41
Sesame	41	0	0	41
Cottonseed	27	0	0	27
Sunflower	27	0	0	27
Cocoa butter	14	0	0	14
Grape Seed	14	0	0	14

FATTY ACID .5 oz. = 1 Tbsp.= ≈14 g.	ALPHA LINOLE NIC (ALA) mg.	EPA mg.	DHA mg.	TOTAL OMEGA 3 mg.
Safflower	13	0	0	13
Coconut	3	0	0	3

26 , 27 , 28

You may notice that our fatty acid chart is much shorter now. That's because only those food sources of Omega 3 polyunsaturated fatty acids are included. We began our work with about 51 fats.

Hemp, flax, and walnuts give us oils that are all high in Omega 3 polyunsaturated fatty acids (PUFAs). It is better to use the seeds or the nuts than commercially prepared oils, because any heat that may be used during any type of processing can ruin many of the health benefits of these oils.

Coconut, safflower, and grape seed oils which are popularly used in preparing many convenience foods have very little of the Omega 3's. They are usually very cheap, too. Not only are they cheap, but grocery stores usually have shelf upon shelf of these types of oils available at very low price points. These oils are sitting in stacks on the store shelves in clear plastic bottles, which exposes these oils to light, encouraging their further degradation.

So it is also important to purchase foods high in Omega 3's in non-transparent containers that protect them. (More on this subject below.) The best and most healthful are organic, packaged in a dark container, and kept in the refrigerator or freezer section at your grocers. And you should store them in your own refrigerator or freezer when you get them home. The best food sources include flax seed, walnuts, and canola. We'll look a lot closer at some details on canola oil latter in this chapter. These delicacies are all best kept in the freezer or under refrigeration to protect their freshness, and allowing them to deliver their goodness to you.

It is also very worthwhile to purchase your nuts and seeds from a natural grocer – and one who stores them under refrigeration or in a freezer. That's because nuts and seeds contain a lot of Omega 3 polyunsaturated fatty acids, which we already know are very delicate. So storing them cold is the best way to assure that the delicate oils in our nuts and seeds remain fresh. And when you get them home, store them in your own freezer as well. Many of us find that we can taste the difference when the oils in these foods are fresh, as well. Maybe you are up for a taste test.

If you have some nuts at home, buy the same type of nuts that have been stored in a cold dark place like a refrigerator or freezer. When you get them home, put them to the taste test so you can compare them for yourself.

For example, if you have some walnuts you purchased from a general grocery store in one of those see-through plastic bags stacked on a shelf exposed to light and room temperature, take one of those walnuts out of the bag for your taste test. Now remove a walnut from the container you just purchased that was stored in a grocer's freezer. Taste the one that was stored in a freezer first, and get a good sense of the aroma, flavor, and texture. Now taste the one you had in your pantry, and get a good sense of its aroma, flavor, and texture. See if you notice a difference in these two nuts.

When nuts and seeds are exposed to heat and light the oils in them begin to deteriorate and become rancid. While those stored in a clear plastic bag on the general shelves of the store may have a good expiration date, their optimal freshness, aroma, and flavor has long departed.

You likely noticed in the Total Omega 3 chart we just looked at that some fish oils are especially high in PUFAs too. Their special goodness deserves more recognition.

Alpha Linolenic Acid (ALA) can be converted by our bodies into EPA and DHA to some minor degree by our livers, but scientists speculate that it happens at only a one to fifteen percent conversion rate. So we might want to look at additional sources to meet our dietary health-building needs. That brings us back to the subject of fish and other seafood, which are the top sources of EPA and DHA, two Omega 3 fatty acids with a great track record in scientific research.

The National Institutes of Health, Office of Dietary Supplements puts out updates for Health Professionals. In their update published on November 21, 2018, they had this to say regarding fish and fish oils:

- "According to both primary and secondary prevention studies, consumption of omega-3 fatty acids, fish, and fish oil reduces all-cause mortality and various CVD outcomes such as sudden death, cardiac death, and myocardial infarction.
- The evidence is strongest for fish and fish oil supplements.
- Fish oils can lower blood triglyceride levels in a dose-dependent manner.
- Omega-3 fatty acids can reduce joint tenderness and need for corticosteroid drugs in rheumatoid arthritis."[29]

Since fish oils can lower blood triglyceride levels in a dose dependent manner, assuring sufficient dietary sources can be considered as a first line health builder. They certainly deserve credit as a simple, natural means to lower triglyceride levels and build cardiovascular health.

And if Omega 3 fatty acids reduce joint tenderness *and* the need for steroid drugs, there is so much we can do on our own on a preventative and natural healing basis.

Rheumatoid arthritis is commonly treated by our physicians with steroids. While many types of insurances may cover this form of treatment, steroids have many negative side effects. Physicians are bombarded by pharmaceutical company reps, and a drug is so much quicker and easier to dispense than is a lesson on the benefits of incorporating Omega 3 fatty acids, including EPA and DHA into our meal patterns.

Fish and fish oils are the top sources of EPA and DHA. Their goodness actually comes to us through the food chain. EPA and DHA are actually formed by *microalgae* ... that are eaten by *phytoplankton* ... that are eaten by *fish*. "When fish consume phytoplankton that consumed microalgae, they accumulate the omega-3s in their tissues."[30] The best dietary sources are *small* fish due to the methyl mercury that accumulates in the larger fish as they grow.

Chicken eggs may also be enriched with EPA and DHA too, through the diets fed to the chickens that lay those eggs. Eggs produced by hens that roam the fields and eat a diet rich in insects and grasses come already complete with natural EPA and DHA. The addition of fish oils to the diets of grain fed hens can increase the amount of EPA and DHA in their eggs. Some consumers may find that this practice leads to a noticeable "fishy" taste to the eggs. You can avoid this by purchasing the eggs of "Free Range" chickens.

Another option might be to skip the entire food chain discussed above, and go directly to the source. You can purchase your own algal, or algae oils to get some EPA and DHA. After all, that's how the fish get theirs. But somehow those fish seem to manage to concentrate the EPA and DHA from the phytoplankton in their diets. We can see from the polyunsaturated fats chart in this book that there is really not very much total polyunsaturated fatty acids in algae oil (only 500 mg. or .0005 g.) in a one tablespoon or 14 g. serving. But even this small amount is still way more than we find in veal or pork fat.

The best seafood dietary sources of EPA and DHA include salmon, sardines, and menhaden. But skip the big fish because of the mercury issue. Remember that the *smaller* fish are the best sources.

And speaking of small fish brings us to the subject of krill. Krill are a very small fish species enjoyed by the whales in our oceans as the majority of their diets. Krill are also at the bottom end of the food chain, close to algae. Krill are also currently being responsibly farmed and harvested for use as a supplement, and sold as krill oil.

A one gram (1,000 mg.) serving of krill oil or two 500 mg. pearls provide about 220 mg. of Omega 3 polyunsaturated fatty acids. This serving provides 120 mg. of EPA and 55 mg. DHA.

We have had much discussion on the oxidation process of fatty acids, and especially omega 3 fatty acids. Krill oil contains a natural anti-oxidant. The 1000 mg. serving discussed above also contains 80 µg. (or micrograms) of astaxanthin a natural component of krill oil, and the magic constituent that prolongs its freshness. Astaxanthin is a powerful anti-inflammatory agent, as it directly lowers our C - reactive protein levels, a biomarker that measures inflammation. If you are considering purchasing an astaxanthin supplement, be sure to read the "Ingredients" label. You want to be sure to get your astaxanthin from *haematococcus pluviaris microalgae*. Some synthetic supplements are also available, made from petrochemical sources.

Other sources of astaxanthin include crayfish, krill, shrimp, trout, and wild caught salmon. Astaxanthin is what creates the red coloring of these marine animals.

Krill oil is a very bioavailable form of polyunsaturated fatty acids. This form of Omega 3's is found deeply embedded in the cell membranes of many of our organs and tissues. Some of the most important are our hearts, the retinas of our eyes, and our nerves.

In November 2018, the journal *Nutrients* published the article "A Comprehensive Review of Chemistry, Sources and Bioavailability of Omega-3 Fatty Acids." The authors of this extensive review point out that, "Krill oil inhibits de novo [a Latin term used to mean "from the beginning"] lipogenesis [conversion to fat deposits], but enhances fatty oxidation [broken down by mitochondria]."[31] Many researchers recommend that these Omega 3's are taken with meals containing fats to be best absorbed. The evening meal may offer the best timing.

Krill oil is not included in the following chart because we would need to consume about 14 g. of it (or about twenty eight 500 mg. pearls) to be able to compare it to the .5 oz. (1 Tbsp. or 14 g.) serving size of the other EPA and DHA food sources. But small amounts of precise fatty acids can be very powerful. We'll be looking closer at just how powerful they can be when we look at trans fats. If you think that just one gram of krill oil is a small amount, trans fats are so powerful that a mere half a gram per serving must bear a health warning on the label of that product. More on that in a bit.

So here is a chart that details some popular dietary sources of EPA and DHA. Keep in mind that we are looking at the oil portion of the fish, or the fat portion of the animal. The serving of each is .5 oz. or 1 Tablespoon or 14 grams.

Figure 8: EPA & DHA FOOD SOURCES

FATTY ACID .5 oz. = 1 Tbsp.= ≈14 g.	EPA mg.	DHA mg.
Fish, salmon	1771	2480
Fish, sardine	1379	1449
Fish, menhaden	1791	1164
Fish, herring	853	572
Fish, cod liver	938	127
Veal fat	2	10
Pork fat	0	7

32

OMEGA 6:3 RATIO

The Omega 6:3 Ratio has a strong basis in scientific research results. The ratio is calculated by dividing the total amount of the greatest one by the total amount of the lesser one. Why would we want to do this? It might just allow us to anticipate how best to address many metabolically affected issues of our health. We looked at some of the work of Artemis Simopoulus earlier when we talked about our natural Omega 6:3 Ratio being 1:1. We're going to look at more of her work now.

The journal of *Biomedicine and Pharmacotherapy* published the research of Artemis Simopoulos of the Center for Genetics, Nutrition and Health in Washington Dc in 2002. The research is titled "The Importance of the Ratio of Omega-6/Omega-3 Fatty Acids." This research is archived in the US National Library of Medicine, National Institutes of Health. We'll detail some of the findings here:

- "In the secondary prevention of cardiovascular disease, a ratio of 4/1 was associated with a 70% decrease in total mortality.

- A ratio of 2.5/1 reduced rectal cell proliferation in patients with colorectal cancer, whereas a ratio of 4/1 with the same amount of omega-3 PUFA had no effect.
- The lower omega-6/omega-3 ratio in women with breast cancer was associated with decreased risk.
- A ratio of 2-3/1 suppressed inflammation in patients with rheumatoid arthritis, and
- a ratio of 5/1 had a beneficial effect on patients with asthma, whereas a ratio of 10/1 had adverse consequences."[33]

This seems to make it pretty clear then that food sources having lower amounts of Omega 6's compared to the amounts of Omega 3's offer the greatest advantage to our health. These studies also indicate that the optimal ratio may vary according to the specific health challenge under consideration.

That leads us to our next goal. We'll detail the Omega 6 to Omega 3 ratio for our group of fats.

The following chart lists our fatty acid food sources alphabetically in the first column. The second column displays the total amount of Omega 6's in these food sources. The third column lists the total amount of Omega 3's in these food sources.

Using this information, we build the important Omega 6:3 "Ratio" of that food, shown in the fourth column. The goal of this chart is to detail the Omega ratio to make this information about these ratios clear for anyone who wants to get back as close as they can to our original Omega 6:3 balance of 1:1, the way nature intended.

The amounts of both Omega 6's and Omega 3's are listed in milligrams (mg.).

NUTRIENT ESSENTIALS

*Note: {Where some foods may have N/A entered in the Ratio column is because those foods contain 0 (zero) amounts of Omega 3 fatty acids. In actuality, no ratio can be calculated for that food. Those food sources that list N/A in the ratio column are included in this chart because some of these are very commonly used as cooking oils. They are included in this chart so you can at least imagine what the Omega 6:3 ratio might look like for these fatty acids, if indeed, they contained any Omega 3's at all. So we can imagine that, for example, Almond oil would have a ratio of 2370:0.} ~ *End of note.

The foods are listed alphabetically. We have 44 fats in this chart because we are including those that only contain Omega 6 fatty acids. We would have only 37 if we left out the fats containing no Omega 3's. All serving sizes are for .5 oz., or 1 Tbsp., or 14 grams of the oil or fat portion only of animal fats:

Figure 9: OMEGA 6:3 RATIOS

FATTY ACID .5 oz. = 1 Tbsp.= ≈14 g.	TOTAL OMEGA 6 mg.	TOTAL OMEGA 3 mg.	OMEGA 6:3 RATIO
Almond	2370	0	N/A
Apricot kernel	3985	0	N/A
Avocado	1754	130	13.1:1
Babassu	220	0	N/A
Bacon grease	1310	129	10.2:1
Beef fat	397	77	5.2:1
Butter	260	168	1.5:1
Canola	2661	1279	2.1:1
Canola for commercial deep frying	1706	200	8.5:1
Corn	7224	157	46:1
Chicken fat	2881	130	19.2:1
Cocoa butter	381	14	27.2:1
Coconut	229	3	76.3:1
Cottonseed	7018	27	260:1

FATTY ACID .5 oz. = 1 Tbsp.= ≈14 g.	TOTAL OMEGA 6 mg.	TOTAL OMEGA 3 mg.	OMEGA 6:3 RATIO
Fish, cod liver	254	1192	1:4.7
Fish, herring	195	1529	1:7.8
Fish, menhaden	452	3158	1:7
Fish, salmon	302	4395	1:14.6
Fish, sardine	513	3008	1:5.9
Flax seed	1900	7640	1:4
Goose fat	1254	64	19.6:1
Grape Seed	9466	14	676:1
Hazelnut	1374	0	N/A
Lamb fat	271	113	2.4:1
Lard	1306	128	10.2:1
Mustard	2146	826	2.6:1
Oat	5315	243	21.9:1
Olive	1318	103	12.8:1
Palm kernel	218	0	N/A
Peanut	4320	0	N/A
Poppyseed	8486	0	N/A
Pork fat	1696	90	18.9:1
Rice bran	4542	218	20.8:1
Safflower	1730	13	131:1
Sesame	5617	41	137:1
Sheanut	666	41	16.2:1
Soybean lecithin	5465	698	7.8:1
Sunflower	5413	27	200:1
Teaseed	3019	95	31.7:1
Tomato seed	6909	313	22.1:1
Turkey fat	2736	179	15.3:1
Veal fat	169	58	2.9:1
Walnut	7194	1414	5.1:1
Wheat Germ	2466	310	8:1

34, 35, 36

We are most affected by the things we do on a regular basis. This includes the foods we eat. When we make a change for the better to some of those things we regularly do, we change a pattern in our lives. As the patterns in our lives change, we do too. A pattern becomes a habit in just a short period of time. So our goal is to look at the little things that can and do make a big difference in our health and in our lives. A little change here and there can make a big impact.

As we become aware of the importance of the balance of our original Omega 6:3 Ratio of 1:1 and how important it may be for us to achieve that balance, it might be wise to review any of our dietary supplements, especially any that are delivered through a gelatin based "pearl" or "soft gel" type of delivery system. This may be particularly true for you if you are experiencing any type of inflammation.

For instance, many brands of supplements for such things as garlic or lutein are found to contain safflower oil listed as the very first "other ingredient." Safflower has an Omega 6:3 Ratio of 131:1.

We now know, after looking at the Omega 6:3 Ratio Chart above, that this means we will need to get 131 times more Omega 3's in order to balance out whatever amount of safflower oil the supplement manufacturer used to fill that "pearl" delivering the garlic or lutein, in order to keep our Omegas in their ideal balance. Different brands may use different filler oils. It might be worth seeking out brands that don't add these oils which are high in Omega 6 fatty acids. There are others available that do not. We vote with our wallets.

Cottonseed oil is pretty bad, at 261:1, nearly two times as bad as safflower. Sunflower oil comes in at 200:1. Sunflower oil is also a very common additive to many pearl type supplements. So it may be highly worthwhile to read the "other ingredients" section of your supplement labels carefully. This way you can select those supplements that do not contain these types of filler oils because they have such high amounts of Omega 6's compared to Omega 3's. And the Omega 6's are directly connected to inflammation.

Peanut oil and poppyseed oil are simply the very worst. They weigh in at 4,320 and 8,486 mg. of total Omega 6's respectively, with no Omega 3's at all to balance them out.

Even bacon grease, butter, and beef fat even have a much healthier Omega 6:3 ratio than safflower, sunflower, or peanut oil, (although bacon grease, butter and beef fat are highly unlikely to be used as fillers to deliver healthy oils in supplement form).

SATURATED FATS

Saturated fats are reputed to drive up our cholesterol levels. These fats are solid at room temperature.

Some obvious sources of saturated fats include red meat, bacon grease or beef fat. Saturated fats are also in prepared baked goods, whole fat dairy products, and coconut oil. The USDA recommends we keep saturated fats to 6% or less of our daily calories. (That comes to about 13 g. per day for a 2000 calorie diet. An avalanche of scientific research is ongoing and has been conducted on saturated fats in the diet.

In a study published in 2016 by the *American Journal of Clinical Nutrition*, researchers reviewed the dietary patterns of fatty acid consumption. Their review included 222,234 adults for over 5 million human years of follow-up. They were wondering if consuming dairy fat might lead to cardiovascular disease. After the researchers studied the dietary data on all these people, the researchers concluded that, "The replacement of 5% of energy intake from dairy fat with an equivalent energy intake from polyunsaturated fat from vegetable sources was associated with 24% reduction in cardiovascular risk."[37] In conclusion, the study authors state that "replacement of animal fats, including dairy fats, with vegetable sources of fats and PUFA's [polyunsaturated fatty acids] may reduce risk of CVD [cardiovascular disease]." [38]

What is somewhat surprising is that a 24% reduction in cardiovascular risk was seen by replacing only 5% of dairy fat with polyunsaturated fats. That's quite a significant impact.

Research in 2015 published by the Journal of Molecular Science states that "Replacing SFAs [Saturated Fatty Acids] with PUFAs [Polyunsaturated Fatty Acids] was inversely associated with the risk of CHD [Coronary Heart Disease]."[39] So once again, replacing saturated fats with polyunsaturated fats lowered the risk of heart disease.

In a 2016 study published by the journal *Diabetes*, researchers tell us that "In humans, high-SFA [Saturated Fatty Acid] consumers, but not high-MUFA [Monounsaturated Fatty Acid] consumers, displayed reduced insulin sensitivity."[40] So diets that are high in saturated fatty acids reduced insulin sensitivity. Diets high in monounsaturated fatty acids did not reduce insulin sensitivity.

Results are hotly debated, as is the benefit vs. detriment of saturated fats of *any* particular type in the diet. Even among research results published as recently as 2019, conflicting evidence continues to exist. Since there is so much conflicting evidence, reading the fine print of research studies can be most valuable.

Earlier studies report that full fat dairy is a powerful detriment to health, yet recent studies (PURE) report that pastured cows roaming the fields grazing on natural grasses produce milk high in Omega 3's as well as vitamins K. These health benefits are only available when the milk from these cows is consumed raw, and not pasteurized. Pasteurization destroys the vitality of many micronutrients. In the case of Omega 3's, heat may turn them into trans fats. Seeking out a local farmer who sells raw milk from pastured cows may be an option you may like to explore.

Scientists do seem to agree, however, that it is best to replace saturated fats, including the popular coconut oil, with polyunsaturated fats. That's because monounsaturated and Omega 3 polyunsaturated fats are proven to reduce inflammation, lower the risk of heart disease and other non-communicable diseases. And as we talked about earlier, it is *only* the polyunsaturated fatty acids that are essential to our lives.

Here is a chart that displays food sources of saturated fatty acids according to the amount of saturated fatty acids they contain. Please notice that the amount of saturated fat these foods contain is measured in *grams*, not milligrams as are the treasured polyunsaturated fats we looked at in earlier charts. This chart displays foods with the greatest amount of saturated fats at the top of the chart. At the bottom of the chart you will find foods with the least amount of saturated fats. Note that we are back up to 51 fatty acids. That's because saturated fats are part of all fatty acid profiles. All of the data here is given for a 1 Tbsp. serving size, or .5 oz. or 14 g.:

Figure 10: SATURATED FATS

Oils, AKA Fatty Acids 1 Tbsp. =.5 Oz. ≈14 g.	Saturated g.
Coconut, virgin	13
Coconut, refined	13
Palm kernel	11.1
Babassu	11.04
Cocoa butter	8.12
Butter, clarified	7.50
Butter	7.17
Palm	6.71
Beef fat	6.37
Sheanut	6.34
Bacon grease	5.03
Lard	5.01
Lamb fat	5.00

Oils, AKA Fatty Acids 1 Tbsp. =.5 Oz. ≈14 g.	Saturated g.
Fish, menhaden	4.14
Fish, sardine	4.07
Chicken fat	3.81
Turkey fat	3.76
Goose fat	3.55
Cottonseed	3.52
Veal fat	3.33
Pork fat	3.11
Fish, cod liver	3.08
Fish, herring	2.90
Teaseed	2.87
Fish, salmon	2.70
Salmon oil	2.70
Rice bran	2.68
Tomato seed	2.68
Oat	2.67
Wheat Germ	2.56
Soybean lecithin	2.04
Corn	2
Peanut	2
Soybean	2
Extra Virgin Olive	1.99
Grape Seed	1.99
Olive	1.86
Poppyseed	1.83
Mustard	1.62
Avocado	1.6
Canola for commercial deep frying	1.38
Walnut	1.24
Almond	1.12
Canola	1.03
Flax seed	1
Hazelnut	1
Hemp, cold pressed	1
Safflower	1.00
Sunflower	1
Apricot kernel	.86
Algae	.500

41, 42, 43

THE DARK SIDE OF FATTY ACIDS

We still have so much research to do. That's why some fatty acids are on the dark side. We'll look at what we do know from scientific studies, and where we can go from here.

Medium chain triglycerides (MCT's) are a naturally occurring small component of virgin coconut and palm kernel oils (they comprise about 14% of these oils). MCT oils are also available as supplements in a concentrated form, as odorless, fractionated, refined oils. The end result, or MCT oil, is a commercially processed product extracted from coconut, and/or palm kernel oil.

We have a history of successfully treating severe childhood epilepsy with medium-chain triglycerides, useful to stop seizures. We also find them to be beneficial to those underweight and other individuals suffering from malabsorption issues.

Some people cannot digest certain foods properly, like wheat and dairy, for instance, which are so very ever-present in many of our refined food products today. For some of these folks, the beauty of MCT oils are that they are digested by the liver, alleviating the body of the need for the pancreatic activity (insulin) required for carbohydrate metabolism. This allows the energy from MCT oils to be more immediately available to our bodies.

MCT oil has become the modern rage, and is promoted by celebrities (many of whom even offer their own brands of these oils for sale) as a safe and easy haven for those primarily seeking weight loss. This is a direct "conflict of interest," and so buyer beware. If this speaks to you, you might look into *"The Complete Guide to Fasting*[44]*"* by Jason Fung and Jimmy Moore.

We just don't have long-term research on people using MCT oils for weight loss. But we do have some recent research on medium chain triglycerides and ketogenic diets using mice and rats as subjects. So we will take a look at some of those.

Using aged rats for subjects, researchers concluded in an April, 2018 study published in the journal *Nutrients*, that " MCFA [medium chain fatty acids] help ß-cells recover from lipotoxic stress by improving mitochondrial function and increasing the expression of genes involved in ß-cell function and insulin biogenesis, such as Glut2, MafA, and NeuroD1 in primary human islets. MCFA offers a therapeutic advantage in the preservation of ß-cell function as part of a preventative strategy against diabetes in at risk populations."[45] This holds hope that there may be help on the horizon for those who are among the "at risk" population for developing diabetes, but please note that the authors do recommend it as part of a *preventive* strategy.

And then, another August, 2018 rodent study published in the journal *Physiology* may raise an alert for those with type 2 diabetes considering the use of a ketogenic diet. This study is aptly titled "Short-term feeding of a ketogenic diet induces more severe hepatic insulin resistance than an obesogenic high-fat diet." The high-fat "obesogenic" diet referred to is considered a typical Western type diet consisting of 60% fat, 20% protein, and 20% carbohydrates. The ketogenic diet referred to was 90% fat. The study authors conclude that, "A glucose challenge reveals that both KD [ketogenic diet] and HFD [high fat Westernized type diet] fed animals are glucose intolerant."[46] Becoming intolerant of glucose may be a seriously overlooked problem. The cost of losing weight on a ketogenic diet may be very great indeed. What happens if you go off of that ketogenic diet of 90% fat? If you have become glucose intolerant, what happens if you ever eat any foods again that contain carbohydrate which converts to glucose during digestion?

These types of research may very well be as valid for humans as they are for rodents. We are certainly much more alike than we are different. After all, both of us (rodents and humans) have pancreases, intestines, and nervous systems. A great blessing to speed our insight is granted by the fact that rodents have a much reduced life-cycle compared to ours. While it would take us maybe twenty five or fifty human life years to experiment with human subjects, the rodents may demonstrate results for us in just a month. The average life of a mouse is just two years, whereas a human can be expected to live for seventy five to eighty years.

With little evidence from long-term human trials, some may accept the data from rodent trials, since we are more alike than different. But this type of data has been long questioned by science and the FDA (food and drug administration), as only human trials were considered valid for human use of a product.

Successful rodent trials may pave the way for human trials, since reliable human trials take a long time. But trans fats were once thought to do great things, too. Only after decades of use we found out the long term effects to our health were devastating.

The standard ketogenic diet is 75% fat, 20% protein, and 5% carbohydrate. Some common side effects are constipation, high cholesterol levels, slowing growth, acidosis, and kidney stones.

And then there are the questionable studies that might be considered to be misleading. Here's one of those: Researchers in Kuwait recruited 83 human subjects to test what they considered a ketogenic diet. The journal *Experimental & Clinical Cardiology* published their study in their fall, 2004 issue. The title of their research is "Long-term effects of a ketogenic diet in obese patients."[47] The study lasted for 24 weeks. That's about six months. Do you think 24 weeks constitutes a long term study?

The researchers report that their subjects' diet consisted of 20-30 g. carbohydrate, 80-100 g. protein, with 20% saturated fat and 80% polyunsaturated and monounsaturated fat. After the first 12 weeks of the study, the carbohydrate content of their diets was increased to 40-50 g. of carbohydrate each day. Do you think this is a ketogenic diet? Can you imagine this as a low-carb diet?

These researchers also included a daily supplement for each of their subjects. This supplement consisted of a capsule weighing in at 45 g. (To put this into perspective, 28 g. is one ounce.)

So these subjects also consumed a specially formulated capsule each day that contained close to two ounces of quite a long list of supplemental micronutrients.

Among the listed micronutrients contained in this daily capsule are lecithin. Lecithin is a fat emulsifier. Our bodies use lecithin to remove excess fats, including triglycerides from our bloodstream. (A common problem with ketogenic diets is high triglyceride levels, leading many to take pharmaceuticals.)

Another important flaw in the design of this study is that it did not have a control group. The results of the study were great, with all subjects losing weight and reflecting much improved blood chemistry. But do you think those capsule ingredients had anything to do with the success of the subjects who participated in this study?

How can we possibly assess the results of the treatment of the subjects without a control group that did not receive the same treatment? Have you ever run the numbers on your own diet?

You should be aware of the pitfalls. While celebrities may promote the use of ketogenic diets, very little, if any warnings are included in their promotional materials regarding these types of diets. It's important to note, for instance, that those who currently hold a diabetes diagnosis, the state of "ketosis," popularly advertised as a cure for all metabolic issues holds the potential to cause "ketoacidosis" and lead to death.

This condition sets up because their bodies do not have enough insulin to break down carbohydrates. So the body breaks down fatty acids instead, resulting in elevated ketone levels (ketosis). Symptoms include excessive thirst, frequent urination, nausea and vomiting, abdominal pain, shortness of breath, tiredness, fruity-scented breath, and confusion.

You should contact your doctor immediately if you're vomiting and unable to keep food or liquids down, if your blood sugar level is higher than your target range and doesn't respond to home treatment, or if your urine ketone level is moderate or high.

You should get emergency help if your blood sugar level is consistently high, 300 mg/dl, if you have ketones in your urine and can't reach your doctor for advice, or if you have a combination of the symptoms of diabetic ketoacidosis like fruity-scented breath, confusion, abdominal pain, excessive thirst, frequent urination, nausea and vomiting, or shortness of breath.

Maybe you or someone you know has jumped onto the ketogenic diet or MCT bandwagon. While some short term studies using human subjects may support the use of MCT's for weight loss, an equal amount of research opposes its' use. And then there are the questionable studies like the one we just looked at.

We still have much research to do. We do know that for an individual with known or even unknown diabetes, a ketogenic diet can quickly lead them from ketosis straight into ketoacidosis, and cause death. Please speak with your physician about your ideas if you have insulin resistance, prediabetes, or type 2 diabetes. Be certain that your physician is knowledgeable in this area, is aware of your condition, and willing to provide the ongoing supervision necessary to guard your health. This is doubly true if you are taking any diabetes medications.

Most diabetes medications are given in dosages based on carbohydrate consumption. When you lower your carbohydrate consumption, if the dosages of these medications are not reduced accordingly, you risk hypoglycemia (low blood sugar).

Symptoms of hypoglycemia include blood sugar levels below 72mg/dl, tiredness, excessive sweating, mental confusion, dizziness, and headache.

And keep in mind that MCT's are a refined oil. Some people find that they just don't get along well with it. Get emergency help if you have signs of an allergic reaction such as hives, difficulty breathing, swelling of the face, lips, tongue, or throat; diarrhea, or stomach pain.

If you are considering ways to lower your cholesterol by using coconut oil, research published in 2018 by the journal *Nutrition*, researchers found that "corn oil lowers plasma cholesterol better than coconut oil."[48]

Please be sure to always eat a lot of vegetables no matter what. Most vegetables are very low in carbohydrates, and most of the carbohydrates they do contain consist of fiber. Fiber delivers many blessings to our bodies as it just naturally traps and removes many of the things our bodies wish to discard. Vegetables bring us micronutrients in their live cells like the chlorophyll they create from the sun, antioxidants, and phytochemicals that keep us young and healthy.

And live foods from the vegetable kingdom also provide fatty acids that are healthful to our bodies without debate. This time we're going to look at the results of a real long-term study. *The Lancet Public Health* published the study "Dietary carbohydrate intake and mortality: a prospective cohort study and meta-analysis" in August 2018.

In this report, the researchers "Studied 15,428 adults for 25 years." The researchers concluded "animal-based low carbohydrate diets should be discouraged. Alternatively, when restricting carbohydrate intake, replacement of carbohydrates with predominantly plant-based fats and proteins could be considered as a long-term approach to promote healthy aging."[49]

Who doesn't want to live a long *healthy* life? Health is the key. The trouble with fad dietary approaches calling for lots of saturated fats and MCT oils is that they haven't been around long enough to give us realistic results based on large groups of humans over long periods of time. So we really don't know what the long term consequences might be for human use.

But we do have recent research about human use of high fat diets. According to the 2018 journal article published in *Oxidative Medicine and Cellular Longevity*, "the HFD [high fat diet] may serve as a stimulus to elevate the systemic inflammatory response in the development of obesity, CVD, diabetes, and cancers."[50] And there is more: "A high-fat diet (HFD) was demonstrated to be a significant risk factor for health…long-term HFD reduced auditory function and promoted age-related hearing loss."[51]

We know that oil of any kind, including MCT oil, has about 120 calories per tablespoon. And adding tablespoons of MCT or coconut oil and butter to our coffee quickly turns a calorie-free beverage into 500 calories.

In the September 2018 issue of the journal *Current Nutrition Report,* we find an article titled "Are We Going Nuts Over Coconut Oil?" The authors say of their research that, "Until the long-term effects of coconut oil on cardiovascular health are clearly established, coconut oil should be considered as a saturated fat and its consumption should not exceed the USDA's daily recommendation (less than 10% of total calorie intake)."[52]

The *American College of Nutrition*, in November 2018, published the article "Health Effects of Coconut Oil – A Narrative Review of Current Evidence." The authors state that, "Limited evidence does not support use for prevention or treatment of Alzheimer's disease, bone loss, or glycemic control. Evidence on weight loss and cardiovascular disease warrants larger clinical intervention studies."[53]

Besides, for some, the negative side effects of adding coconut oil or MCT's to their diet are just too hard to take. Bloating, joint pain, inflammation, gout, bald patches, and even "electrical" cramps and neurological issues are reported. The symptoms left within a few days after coconut oil or MCT's were abandoned from their diets.

Some of us may just be genetically different in our capacity to utilize some types of oils. It is suggested that some of us may be missing a certain gene. As artificial intelligence participates to a greater extent in our healthcare system, we may locate the precise gene involved. Sequencing the genomes of those facing health challenges may require the inspection of 5 million pieces of data. With Artificial Intelligence we can accomplish this using machine-learning algorithms to distill those genomes pertinent to the root cause of any health challenge. This will open a door to a new treatment model directly addressing genetic variances. That's when it does in fact become available on a large scale.

Many may experience an inability to digest coconut oil, or may find they are just allergic to it. For those with an allergy to coconuts, coconut oil can cause havoc in the body. This is also as true for MCT oil derived from coconut oil as it is for just plain coconut oil itself. If this sounds like your allergic situation, you should also avoid any skin creams or shampoos containing coconut oil as well. Reading the ingredient label on any personal care products is very important for your health and wellbeing.

TRANS FATS

The top four most popular oils used today are canola, corn, palm, and soybean. These are all typically refined oils, like the ones you see in clear plastic bottles piled high on the shelves at your general grocers. These refined oils all contain a certain amount of *trans* fats, or "refined fats."

Let's look at how the refining process of these oils works. During the "refining" process, seeds are pressed, heated, and treated to some amount of hexane gas to extract extra oils. But we also get hexane gas from gasoline fumes.[54] While this hexane gas is thought to be safe at the levels that remain in any of our refined oils, each of us can decide for themselves whether or not we want our oils spiked with the stuff. The final step in the refining process is deodorizing. Deodorizing is done to remove much of the flavor of the oil to suit the reportedly preferred tastes of the consumer.

So you can see, most of the oils sold in supermarkets already have some amount of trans fats just because of the way the oils are extracted from their plant material, and deodorized, even if they are not specifically labeled as "refined." Then these oils sit on the shelves of grocers in clear containers where they are exposed to light, causing further damage.

These oils didn't start out as trans fats. And trans fats were not *added* to these oils. The heat used during the refining process can turn some of the delicate healthful Omega's they contain into trans fats. Some foods like whole milk dairy products and beef just naturally contain some trans fats, so it may be hard to totally avoid them. But the trans fats created by processing or "refining" vegetable oils are unnecessary. And they can be avoided.

Partially hydrogenated (or trans) fats received analysis as long ago as 1993. Walter Willet and a team of researchers brought this to light in a report funded and published by the *National Institutes of Health*, in 1993.

After carefully examining the *Nurse's Health Study* data (covering the eating habits of more than 85,000 participants) for over a period of eight years, Walter Willets' team pointed out, "Our findings must add to concern that the practice of partially hydrogenating vegetable oils to produce solid fats may have reduced the anticipated benefits of substituting these oils for highly saturated fats, and instead contributed to the occurrence of CHD."[55]

Since we are sorting out our fats, we can look at a basic chart of those trans fats. While there are few, their reach into our food supply is great. We will look at a simple chart of the four of them which highlight the major sources in our diets. These fats are listed by those with the most trans fats at the top of the chart. Please notice that the amount of trans fats in them is listed in grams (g) rather than milligrams (mg.) This is in contrast to the milligrams (mg.) used in measuring our polyunsaturated fats:

Figure 11: TRANS FATTY ACIDS

Oils, AKA Fatty Acids 1 Tbsp./.5 Oz./ ≈14 g.	Trans fat g

Canola for commercial deep frying	3.67	56
Veal fat	0.45	
Pork fat	.09	
Canola	.06	

DETAILS OF TRANS FATS

Ingredient labels mentioning partially hydrogenated vegetable oils are a tip-off that this is the type of oil (fat) in the product. Trans fats raise harmful LDL cholesterol and triglyceride levels. They also lower our helpful HDL levels, extending an invitation to clogged arteries and heart disease. Our bodies just don't seem to know what to do with these trans fats. They are unnatural, and so they are not native to the human diet. And they were not even in existence one hundred years ago.

Even small amounts of trans fats contribute to insulin resistance, increasing the risk for type 2 diabetes. Trans fats also cause inflammation, linked to heart disease, diabetes, stroke and many other chronic non-communicable disease conditions.

Trans fats have long been used in commercial deep frying operations because they can be re-used many times before becoming rancid. Good for the profit of the commercial operation, but not good for us, the consumers of their products. Even in an amount as low as 2% of our daily calories, trans fats raise our risk of heart disease by about 25%.

Canola oil, often considered a healthy monounsaturated fatty acid, is usually treated at high temperatures, causing partial hydrogenation, as in trans fats. Over 90% of canola oil is already genetically modified. Have you ever heard of a canola plant? There isn't one. Canola oil comes from the genetically modified *rapeseed* plant. Then it is refined for human use, because of the naturally high content of Omega 3 fatty acids, which would smell bad when exposed to oxygen and heated. The deodorizing process used during refining turns some 20% of "canola" oils' once healthful Omega 3's into trans fats.

In 2018, the *British Medical Journal (BMJ)* employed a group of scientists to conduct a scientific review of medical research on fats for public health recommendations. The researchers had this to say: "For cardiovascular health, substantial evidence supports the importance of the type of fat consumed, not total fat intake, and the elimination of industrially produced trans fats."[57]

Any ingredient label that includes the words "partially hydrogenated" is telling you there are trans fats in the product. This is true even if the front label on the package says the product contains NO trans fats.

They can make this claim -- and they do -- because the laws allow them to do so. The FDA requires that only products with more than .5 g. of trans fats per serving (a serving size is 1 Tbsp. or 14 g.) to disclose that the product contains trans fats on the ingredient list.

That's because the FDA designates a serving of .5 g. of trans fats as *generally recognized as safe (GRAS)*. We, the people, are left to judge for ourselves, just how much of this poison really is safe.

Let's take a closer look at that because .5 grams is such small amount. Just how small is .5 gram? It takes 28 grams to make one ounce, so one gram = 1/28 oz. Then ½ of 1 gram is 1/56 of an ounce. That means that just a few drops may bring us to our daily limit of what is considered *generally recognized as safe*. For some oils, that amount could even be even less. The point is that we are looking at such a small amount of a substance. The amount is so small in fact, that we can measure it by drops, not mouthfuls. And that is the truth about all of the fats in our lives. A little goes a long way.

Scientific research has revealed that trans fats are so bad for our health that they have been banned in the U.S. So they are being "phased out" of commercial cooking processes. But those products that are already manufactured are being allowed to wait on store shelves for purchase until their presence in our food supply is finally depleted.

And while we have known about the problems caused by trans fats since Walter Willett's research was released in 1993, "The FDA agreed in May 2018 to give companies one more year to find another ingredient for enhancing product flavors or to grease industrial baking pans. Also, while new products can no longer be made with trans fats, they will give foods already on the shelves some time to cycle out of the market."[58]

So in the meantime, these things may be lurking on the shelves at our grocers, just waiting for the unwary shopper to pop them into their grocery carts and take them home to love. That leaves it up to you, the savvy consumer. These foods have a long shelf life, so who knows when we will finally be rid of them? And after all, we've known they were bad for us for a long time. We've already had 25 years, since the publication of Walter Willet's research to clean this up. But have we cleaned it up?

What happens if an unsuspecting person eats several servings each day of foods that contain just a little bit (.5 g., the generally recognized as safe amount) of these partially hydrogenated vegetable oils or trans fats? This, of course, could double, triple, or even quadruple the consumption of these trans fats to unhealthy levels and assert a major negative impact on their health.

Some things that are likely to contain partially hydrogenated vegetable oils or trans fats include coffee creamers, frozen pizza crusts, microwave popcorn, commercially prepared baked goods and frostings that contain "shortening" of any kind (whatever that really is), refrigerated doughs for muffins, cookies, and pizzas; potato, corn, and tortilla chips, and any foods that are cooked by deep frying methods. Remember, we are "using these things up" as they diminish from our food supply.

As of April 2018 the USDA Nutrient database reports that a serving McDonald's® French fries continue to come with trans fats.[59]

Burger King® French fries also include trans fats. But this, in both of these -- and many other cases -- may be due to the naturally occurring trans fats caused by using some amount of innocent polyunsaturated fats in cooking oil recipes -- heated to the extreme temperatures of deep frying for long periods of time, or refining. Not an insect on the face of the earth will eat any of this stuff.

And oils that have been subjected to the refining process are sitting on the shelves at our grocers. They already contain some amount of these trans fats created during the refining process.

And finally, the virtue of refined, partially hydrogenated oils is that they increase the shelf life of those foods that contain them. Having products that can last a lifetime means that there is little waste to be discarded due to spoilage, as is the case with natural foods.

So the question must be asked, and perhaps you wonder, too: How great of a stockpile of these foods do we really have in storage? As we ponder the scope of this stockpile, we may wonder if some of these may even be handed down to the next generation -- or even two. Or perhaps they may one day be discovered among the fossilized remains of our society by our descendants in a thousand years from now. And those trans fatty acid laced foods may very well still be "fresh" enough to eat....

PROTEIN

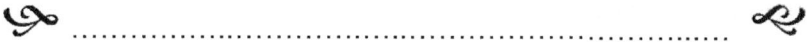

My Plate guidelines recommend that most adults consume about 5 to 6 oz. (150 – 180 g.) of protein (AKA amino acids) each day. For most of us, this is about a one inch thick slice about the size of the palm of our hand. In this chapter we will look at the essential amino acids as well as the amounts of protein we get from different food groups.

While protein-based products like "chicken nuggets" contain some protein, they are typically dipped into a white flour based batter that is *not* protein. A quick review of the nutrition information on the label shows that a 3 oz. serving of one chicken nugget product has 13 g. of protein, but it is wrapped in 18 g. of a carbohydrate based batter. So this product is actually more carbohydrate than it is protein. We will be looking at this situation much closer when we get into GRAINS.

We require protein to build our bodies, but our biological requirement is actually for the amino acids that protein provides. Both animal *and* vegetable (plant) proteins are made up of about 20 amino acids. All protein foods, from both animal (except for gelatin) and plant sources contain some of each amino acid.

ESSENTIAL AMINO ACIDS

There are nine amino acids that are not synthesized by our bodies. These amino acids are considered essential, because they must be consumed by us as part of our diets.

The nine essential amino acids are: histidine, isoleucine, leucine, lysine, methionine, phenylalanine, threonine, tryptophan, and valine. These *nutrient essentials* are listed alphabetically in the following chart. The U.S. recommended daily allowances (USRDA) for each amino acid is included, and works on a sliding scale. The way it works is that for every 2.2 pounds (1 Kg) of body weight, we are advised to include the following amounts (shown in the middle column of the following chart) in our meals:

Figure 12: ESSENTIAL AMINO ACIDS USRDA + FUNCTION

ESSENTIAL AMINO ACID	USRDA	USES IN OUR BODIES
Histidine	14 mg.	Maintains Myelin sheath (protects nerve cells); produces histamine, vital to immune response, digestion, sexual function, and "wake-sleep" cycle.
Isoleucine	19 mg.	Concentrated in muscle tissue; important for hemoglobin production, energy regulation, and immune function.
Leucine	42 mg.	Muscle repair, protein syntheses; helps regulate blood sugar, produces growth hormones, and stimulates wound healing,
Lysine	38 mg.	Plays a major role in hormone and enzyme production, protein syntheses, energy production, collagen, elastin and absorption of calcium.
Methionine	Plus cysteine, a non-essential amino acid, 19 mg.	Necessary for tissue growth, metabolism and detoxification; absorption of zinc (important for healing) and selenium.
Phenylalanine	Plus tyrosine, a	Key player in the structure and function of proteins, enzymes, and

ESSENTIAL AMINO ACID	USRDA	USES IN OUR BODIES
	non-essential amino acid, 33 mg.	other amino acids. Precursor for the neurotransmitters dopamine, epinephrine, norepinephrine and tyrosine.
Threonine	20 mg.	Major part of structural proteins such as collagen and elastin in our skin and connective tissues. Plays a major role in metabolism and immune function.
Tryptophan	5 mg.	Precursor to the neurotransmitter serotonin which regulates mood, appetite, mood, and sleep. Maintains proper nitrogen balance.
Valine	24 mg.	Helps stimulate muscle growth and regeneration. Involved in energy production.

60 61 62 63 64 65 66 67 68 69

Our bodies are clever chemists as they busily match, and re-match; use and re-use these essential amino acid components in various combinations to build whatever our bodies may need on a daily basis. This is the economy of protein digestibility. Even when we are done growing to adulthood, our bodies still need a continual supply of protein for re-building and repair as life goes on and for the life long production of our hair and nails.

All amino acids have a function, and each of them fulfill a need. While we just looked at the essentials in the previous chart, there are other amino acids with major significance as well, and one of these is glycine.

Glycine is an oddball amino acid. It is the smallest, and simplest of all. Glycine is achiral, meaning that it is symmetrical. It's very involved in the production of DNA, phospholipids, and in the release of energy. To that end, it is needed to produce glutathione, an antioxidant that helps protect cells against the damage of oxidative stress.

Glycine is the main amino acid in collagen, which provides strength to our muscles, cartilage, bones, ligaments, and skin. If you don't get enough glycine, your body may not be able to produce enough glutathione or the amino acid creatine, which provides energy for our muscles.

Creatine directs the recycling of adenosine triphosphate (ATP, the energy exchange of our cells, primarily in our muscles and brain tissue. It's a very popular supplement used by body-builders and other athletes. Most people get enough in their meal plans by eating seafood and red meat.

You may notice another effect of creatine. It helps you have a good night of sleep by lowering your bodies' core temperature and also has a calming effect.

Excess amino acids that aren't used by our bodies are easily discarded in our urine, converted to carbohydrate, or stored as fat.

NUTS AND SEEDS

We also get a good amount of protein from nuts, seeds, grains, and legumes (pulses). Our nuts, seeds, grains, and legumes (pulses) come with some amount of phytic acid, also called *phytates*. The phytates envelope micronutrients, making them less bioavailable to our bodies. These phytates may not be a problem for a cow, because cows have four stomachs, one just suited for this. But humans have only one stomach, and lacks the needed phytase, a digestive enzyme used to break down those resistant phytates that make some of the nutrients less available to us.

But there is a way to deal with these phytates. We can break through their boundaries and increase the amount of protein and fiber in the foods that are wrapped in them. This method also causes a decrease in the amount of carbohydrate in these foods as well. We can use the simple technique known as germination to achieve these goals. Germination, also known as "sprouting" is a powerful force in nature. Soaking in water our seeds, grains, and legumes is how we encourage germination.

A tiny seed absorbs moisture to soften its' endosperm for absorption by its germ. The germ portion of the seed sends forth a tiny root to absorb even more water and nutrients for the further growth of the seed. As the seed is further nourished, the germ sends out infant leaves called cotyledons that reach for the sun and create chlorophyll. These cotyledons are nourished from the endosperm portion of the seed until the root is able to maintain the growth of the infant plant. Then the tiny plant grows to maturity. Unless we intercept this process.

We intercept the process when we add the sprouts with their infant cotyledons and roots to our salads, smoothies, or baked goods. Just imagine all the life we are adding to our food when we allow our seeds to sprout before we eat them. In February, 2015, the journal of *Food Science Technology*, published an article titled, "Reduction of phytic acid and enhancement of bioavailable micronutrients in food grains." The researchers in this study concluded that sprouting "reduces phytic acid content by up to 40 %."[70]

Not only are we adding more life to our foods, we add more nutrients as well. You might be wondering just how much these nutrients might be increased by sprouting. The journal of *Food Science Technology* published another article in October, 2015, that gives us more information. The article is titled, "Sprouting characteristics and associated changes in nutritional composition of cowpea (Vigna unguiculata)." While the article is mainly concerned with the researchers' work with cowpeas, they also review the research of other scientists in their article, giving us a bit more information. Here is a summary of what the researchers report:

- "There was significant increase in crude protein after sprouting in all genotypes.
- 19.15 % increase in crude protein content of cowpea [aka black eyed pea] after 28 h of sprouting.
- Significant increase in crude fibre [fiber] was observed after sprouting. where 20 to 24 % increase has been reported after sprouting cowpea.
- 44 % decrease in fat content in sesame seeds after 4 days of sprouting.
- Carbohydrate content of sprouted cowpea was significantly decreased from their raw counterparts.
- There were significant improvement in IVPD [in-vitro (in our bodies) protein digestibility] by 17.00 and 20.80 % when period of sprouting increased from 48 to 60 and 60 to 72 h, respectively.
- Present study shows that sprouting is an effective method for removing anti-nutritional factors in cowpea without application of heat processing methods, which may reduce content of heat sensitive nutrients."[71]

So if you give these seeds a chance at life, they will reward you with about 20% more protein and fiber, and a significant (although the study authors offer no specific measurement) reduction in carbohydrate. Plus, soaking them for three days improves the bioavailability of their protein.

Nuts are very high in fats, and as we talked about earlier, should be stored in a freezer to protect their delicate nutrients. Many have several times as much fat as they do protein, so depending on your goals you might keep this in mind when making your selections.

While many nuts have a glycemic index of 0, others do not. If you are dealing with any level of insulin resistance, selecting from among those nuts with a GI of 0 will keep your blood sugar levels stable. And although we just learned that sprouting reduces carbohydrate content, the extent of that carbohydrate reduction is not quantified. Using calculations that keep you on the side of low glycemic index and low glycemic load may reward with stable blood sugar levels. If you are interested in learning more about using glycemic index and glycemic load for blood sugar control, please see my book *"Cheat Sheet Simply for CA, UK, or USA Foods,"* for country specific scientifically tested foods.

The following chart displays nuts and seeds in their typical serving sizes, and in alphabetical order according to the name of the nut or seed. (1.76 oz. = 50 g.; 1 oz. = 28 g.) The serving sizes are small because nuts and seeds are nutrient dense, high in calories, protein, fiber, and fats, meaning that a little goes a long way toward filling you up and keeping you satisfied.

Figure 13: NUTS & SEEDS MACRONUTRIENTS

NUT/SEED	OZ.	CAL	PROTEIN	CARBS	FIBER	FAT
Almonds	1.76	298	11	11	6	25
Cashews	1.76	281	10	14	2	22
Chia seeds, raw	1	138	5	12	10	9
Filberts/Hazelnuts	1.76	314	7	8	5	4.8
Macadamia	1.76	359	4	7	4	38
Peanuts	1.76	284	13	8	4	25
Pecans	1.76	340	5	7	5	36

NUTRIENT ESSENTIALS

NUT/SEED	OZ.	CAL	PROTEIN	CARBS	FIBER	FAT
Pepitas	1.76	266	15	5	3	23
Pistachios	1.76	280	10	14	5	5
Sesame seeds	1.76	286	9	12	6	25
Sunflower seeds	1.76	284	12	10	5	25
Pumpkin seeds	1.76	320	18	6	4	28
Walnuts	1.76	334	8	7	4	33

72

VEGETABLES

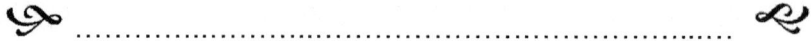

You may be aware that many foods in the vegetable family contain a high percentage of protein. It's not surprising that we may wonder whether vegetables really do provide enough protein that we can actually count on them as a good source for our protein needs.

As human beings, we have a symbiotic relationship with plants. Our lives depend on them. The oxygen we need to breathe to live comes from plants, while the carbon dioxide plants need to live is created in human beings as we exhale. Our relationship with plants really is the perfect partnership for life.

Over the past half a decade, modern food manufacturing practices have grown exponentially. They have made highly processed food products increasingly available in ever-expanding numbers of creative options designed to intervene in our natural relationship with plants. Our waistlines have grown, and our health has suffered in proportion to the amount of these foods we have included in our diets. It's no wonder that our health is effected by these practices. Refined, processed foods have lost many of their micronutrients and phytochemicals that our bodies need in order to maintain a healthy mind and body.

But we can turn the tide on the food manufacturing giants by returning to our natural diet of eating unrefined vegetation products. And it is worth it no matter where we are in our quest to improve our health. In a 2018 study published by the medical journal *Oxidative Medicine and Cellular Longevity* the authors state that "high intakes of fruits and vegetables significantly decreased energy consumption [calories], waist circumference, body weight, and sagittal abdominal diameter in overweight and obese men and women."[73]

The study authors continue on the benefits of these living foods, "Fruits and vegetables not only reduce obesity, CVD, and diabetes but they also inhibit several cancers, demonstrating the numerous functional potentials of fruits and vegetables. Epidemiological studies have shown an inverse relationship between fruit and vegetable intakes and cancer risks such as colon, breast, and prostate cancers. This suppressive effect was mainly observed in cruciferous and green-yellow vegetables."[74] As you can see, this research reported results far beyond controlling expanding waistlines.

Some of our most popular cruciferous vegetables include broccoli, cabbage, Brussels sprouts, arugula, bok choy, collard greens, kale, kohlrabi, and many other similar green leafy vegetables.

Below is a little chart covering about 50 of our most popular vegetables. They are listed here in alphabetical order. Most serving sizes in the chart are about 4 ¼ ounces (120 g.), or the typical serving size of that food. All gram measures of protein, carbs, and fiber are rounded into even numbers.

{*Note: Wheat grass is marked with an asterisk (*). This is because the USDA Nutrient Database does not provide an exact search result for that particular food. There are several proprietary powdered formulations that contain wheat grass, as well as proprietary beverages listed in the database.

Many local health-food type stores carry an organic, pure wheat grass powder. The information in the vegetable chart below is taken from a container of pure organic wheat grass powder. You might add this to your favorite smoothie recipe or simply dissolve in water. There are also many grocers that carry live, organic wheat grass. In my travels, I have found it at Albertson's, Meijer's, Natural Grocers Vitamin Cottage, and Sprouts Farmer's Market.

If you are keen on live wheat grass, you may like to grow your own. Organic wheat grass seeds are available with other vegetable seeds for your gardening fun at some locations.

Or, if you purchase a flat of live wheat grass from a local grocer, you can extend the life of your wheat grass. Simply remove it from the container, pop it into a gardening pot (with holes in the bottom for drainage) that you have filled three quarters full with a good gardening soil and place it outside. Be sure to keep the soil moist. This way you may harvest well over a month of clippings from your modest investment. } ~ *End of note.

Ounce for ounce, most vegetables are low in calories, carbohydrate and fats and high in fiber, except for potatoes. Potatoes are so high in carbohydrate that they are grouped with processed grains in some countries. Potatoes are included with the rest of our vegetables in this chart in order to make it easier to compare all of our most popular vegetables.

In the chart below we can see how many calories, how much protein, carbohydrate, fiber, and fat are in a typical serving of these raw vegetables. The vegetables are listed in this chart in alphabetical order. The serving sizes shown are measured in ounces. If you measure in grams, please refer to the chart in the back of the book.

Figure 14: VEGETABLES MACRONUTRIENTS

VEGETABLE	OZ.	CAL	PROTEIN	CARBS	FIBER	FAT
Artichoke	4.23	23	2.5	13	6	0
Arugula	4.23	30	3.24	4	2	1

NUTRIENT ESSENTIALS

VEGETABLE	OZ.	CAL	PROTEIN	CARBS	FIBER	FAT
Asparagus	4.23	20	2.75	5	3	0
Beet greens	4.23	26	2.75	12	3	0
Bell pepper	4.23	22	1.48	11	2	0
Bok Choy	4.23	17	1.48	7	1	0
Broccoli	4.23	41	3.38	8	3	0
Cabbage	4.23	30	1.6	7	3	0
Carrots	4.23	49	1	12	3	0.29
Cauliflower	4.23	30	2.4	6	2	0.34
Celery	4.23	17	0.86	4	2	0.2
Collard greens	4.23	38	3.78	6	5	0.73
Cucumber	4.23	18	0.81	4	1	0.13
Dandelion greens	4.23	54	3.38	11	4	0.84
Eggplant	4.23	30	1.22	7	4	0.22
Garlic	0.99	42	2	9	1	0.6
Ginger root	0.99	22	1	5	1	0.21
Grape leaves	2.12	56	3.36	10	7	1.26
Green beans	4.23	37	2.29	8	4	0.26
Green Leaf Lettuce	5.29	22	2	4	2	0.22
Jicama	4.23	46	0.86	11	6	0.11
Kale	4.23	42	3.65	11	2	1.79
Kohlrabi	4.23	32	2.13	7	4	0.12
Leek	4.23	73	1.88	17	2	0.36
Mushrooms, white	4.23	26	3.64	4	1	0.41
Mustard greens	4.23	32	3.6	7	9	0.5
Nopal (prickly pear cactus)	4.23	49	1	11	4	0.61
Okra	4.23	40	2.41	8	4	0.23
Olives, plain	4.23	168	0	7	4	18

VEGETABLE	OZ.	CAL	PROTEIN	CARBS	FIBER	FAT
Onion	4.23	48	1.38	11	2	0.12
Parsnips	2.82	32	1	14	4	0.08
Potato, baked russet	5.29	89	3	26	2.1	0
Potato, sweet, baked	5.29	135	3	31	5	.23
Potato, yam, average	5.29	174	2	42	6	0.23
Radicchio	4.23	28	1.72	5.38	1	.30
Radish	1.06			1	1	
Spinach	5.29	34	4.29	4	3	0.58
Swiss chard	4.23		3	4	2	
Tomatillo	4.23	38	1	7	2	1.22
Tomato	4.23	22	1	5	1	0.24
Turmeric powder	.99	87	2.87	19	6	.91
Watercress	4.23	13	3	2	1	0.2
Wheatgrass* powder, organic, dry	.33	30	3	6	3	0
Zucchini	4.23	25	3	4	1	0.48

75

LEGUMES

Another vegetable food group, legumes, also provide high amounts of protein, and may be prominent among your choices. Legumes are considered to provide about 50% of the protein that animal sources do, according to MyPlate guidelines. So for an ounce of protein, you would eat two ounces of legumes, according to these guidelines. But as you will see in the Legume chart, below, some beans fall far short of this general guideline. Different types of beans also contain different amounts of carbohydrate. If you are counting carbs, you'll want to take the carbohydrate content in your beans into your account.

It is interesting to note that the number of carbs in each serving of legumes are as low as 15 and as high as 39. It is also interesting to note that the amount of fiber varies from 9 to 16 g. All of these legumes have a low glycemic index (GI) of 55 or less. Beans (legumes) also have GI values from as low as 10 up to 42. All of them are low GI food choices that bring a lot of fiber to your plate. But be sure to measure your portion sizes for glycemic load (GL).

It's important to eat foods that have a low glycemic index, or low GI. In January, 2018, the journal *Oxidative Stress and Cellular Longevity* published the article "Nutrients and Oxidative Stress: Friend or Foe?" Researchers concluded that "chronic consumption of high GI foods may cause oxidative stress via the formation of free radicals that are capable in destroying biological molecules and initiate abnormal cell growth through gene mutation."[76]

Free radicals are extremely volatile molecules because they are missing a partner electron that would have given them stability. Since they are missing an electron, these molecules are free to roam and hook up with molecules in our bodies where they don't belong. As these free radical molecules go scavenging around among our healthy molecules they cause destruction and the growth of abnormal cells, and even mutations in our genetic material. Oxidative stress is what happens when these molecules that are missing a matching electron (free radicals) over-power the healthy cells in our bodies' natural anti-oxidant system.

Legumes provide a healthy alternative to processed refined grain containing foods. Legumes (beans, or pulses) can handily replace many nutritionally depleted ingredients, such as flour, when building many recipes. When they are boiled, rinsed, drained, and pureed, they make a nutritious, healthy thickener for any sauce or soup that puts any refined flour to nutritional shame.

They also make a superb cake or muffin batter that bakes up moist, tender, low glycemic, and loaded with protein and fiber. For a few recipe ideas, see my book "Are You Sweet Enough Already ? "

And you'll see in the following chart that legumes contain a lot of fiber. Legumes are also associated with a 35% lower adiposity-related cancer rate, thanks to the work of the fiber they contain.

A five and a quarter oz. serving (just over half a cup) is the average serving size. All legumes (pulses) in the chart below are presented in a five and a quarter oz. (or 150 g.) serving. This way you can compare them ounce for ounce to each other.

After this one note, we will look at the chart.

{* Note: The chart below includes entries for unsweetened carob and cocoa powders. The amounts listed are meant to be helpful as you might compare the nutrients in one to the other. These powders are created from grinding these beans and often used when creating dessert recipes. In the case of these two beans, you are not expected to eat 5 ¼ ounces at one serving. These are the amounts meant to be used in entire recipes. So if you are adding one of these powders to one of your recipes, simply add the total amount of each macronutrient to your total recipe ingredient calculations.

For instance, if you want to know how many calories, protein, or carbs one of these two ingredients (carob or cocoa powder) add to each serving, just divide the amount of that ingredient by the number of servings your recipe provides. The same is true of any ingredient you may choose to use in any recipe.} ~ *End of note.

The typical serving size for any of these different legumes (beans, or pulses) is about 5 ¼ ounces (or 150 g.), with the exception of carob or cocoa as we discussed earlier.

Figure 15: LEGUMES/PULSES MACRONUTRIENTS

LEGUME	OZ.	CAL	PROTEIN	CARBS	FIBER	FAT
Black beans, boiled	5.29	198	13	35	13	1
Carob powder, unsweetened *	5.29	350	10	130	70	0
Cocoa powder, unsweetened *	5.29	350	30	90	60	20
Fava/broad beans	5.29	138	8	24	5	1
Garbanzo/Chickpeas, boiled	5.29	165	11	29	8	1
Haricot / Navy beans, boiled	5.29	207	11	34	9	9
Kidney beans, boiled	5.29	210	11	39	15	1
Lentils, cooked	5.29	182	12	31	9	1
Lima beans, boiled	5.29	184	10	35	8	0
Pinto beans	5.29	184	10	35	8	0
Soybean sprouts	5.29	171	10	30	8	1
Soybeans (edamame)	5.29	177	19	14	4	11
Split peas	5.29	212	19	17	6	10
Tofu	5.29	174	13	31	13	13

77

GRAINS

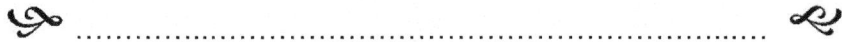

G rains are given an entire section for MyPlate. They are given their own category, much as vegetables, protein, and fruit. We have two types of grains to consider. There are Whole Grains, and there are Refined (or processed) Grains. MyPlate guidelines recommend that we include 50% of each variety, whole grains and refined grains when we build our plates. We'll look at whole grains first, because they are the grains that build our health.

Whole grains are those grains just as they came off the stalk. You can tell whole grains from refined grains because whole grains look just like grains -- because they are. Rye kernels are whole grains; wheat kernels are whole grains. These whole kernel grains have about 100% more bran and germ than any of their refined byproducts. Plus these Whole Grains are loaded with a lot of other nutrition we'll get to in a minute.

It's no wonder that we are encouraged to eat whole grains. A large scale analysis of many scientific studies was published by the journal *Nutrients* in 2017, titled "Whole grain intake and glycaemic control in healthy subjects." Scientists researched and compared the health of populations who eat refined grains to the health of populations who eat whole grains. They report that there is a "decreased risk of CVD, type 2 diabetes, metabolic syndrome, and cancer associated with increased intake of WG [Whole Grain] foods."[78]

Scientists have studied the grain dietary patterns of large populations over the course of many years. The *British Medical Journal* published a study in 2018 titled "Dietary carbohydrates: roll of quality and quantity in chronic disease." The authors report direct "cause and effect" results in the health of many of these populations. Scientists further find that refined grain intake is actually "causally related to the development of type 2 diabetes, coronary heart disease, and perhaps obesity."[79]

But this is comparing whole grain consumption to the consumption of refined grains. Just lowering our chances of CVD, type 2 diabetes, metabolic syndrome, and cancer may be a nice motivating force for choosing whole grains instead of refined grains as our preferred dietary practice.

When we look at filling such a large portion of our ideal plates with "whole grains," what we are looking at are these whole grains that are complete with their entire original "packaging." The original "packaging" of any grain includes the bran (outer-most shell) and the germ (innermost portion), as well as the endosperm (the largest component, nested between the bran and the germ) portion of the grain. The nutrient dense germ and bran factors are stripped away when a grain becomes "refined," leaving only the endosperm portion to be milled into flour. The original packaging is what delivers all of the *synergistic* vitamins B, and all of the omega 3 and 6 lipids naturally present that complete the entire whole grain. We're going to look at that a little closer now.

ESSENTIAL VITAMINS B

Synergistic means that all vitamins B work together. It means that the combined action of all of the vitamins B work -- with each other -- to enhance our health. Synergistic means that their combined action is greater than the action of any individual part, or any specific B vitamin. Or even any specific combination of a couple of vitamins B. And that takes us to the refined grains that are so prevalent in our society today.

Refined grains weren't so popular fifty years ago, but then again, neither was obesity, insulin resistance, or many of the other chronic noncommunicable diseases that are so rampant in our world today.

According to the *National Institutes of Health*, in 1985, our diets included a whopping 287 g. of carbs each day for males, and 177 carbs a day for females. The "Food Pyramid" scheme had carbohydrates as its' base. That pyramid held that we should eat some eight to eleven servings of grain each day, with photos of bread, cereal, pasta, and rice. We're doing a lot better now, with our MyPlate allocations. But do we really need all that grain? And what on earth is the good of refined grains of any type?

Dr. Joel Fuhrman details the epic proportion of this situation in his book *"Fast Food Genocide -- How Processed Food is Killing Us and What We Can do about it."*[80]

Manufacturers often add riboflavin, thiamin, folic acid, and maybe some iron to their refined grain end-products (such as wheat or white flour) used to create bakery products like wheat or white bread, donuts, cookies, chips, bakery made or boxed cakes & mixes and other flour-based products. That is after they have removed most of the nourishment our bodies really need, like the nourishment naturally occurring in the germ and bran portions of the whole grains, because these would quickly spoil.

But the few select vitamins B the manufacturers add just confuses our bodies, since they do not add the entire group of essential vitamins B that were part of that natural grain before they took hold of it. Just adding a few of these vitamins B leaves our bodies without the other vitamins B that our bodies need for the synergistic actions involved in building our health.

There are essential vitamins B, much as there are essential fatty acids and essential amino acids. All essential nutrients are those that we must get from our diet. Our bodies need them to live.

These essentials are indispensable.

There are eight essential vitamins B that we must get from our meal patterns. Our bodies can use these to make other vitamins B. Here is a little chart that shows which ones are indispensable and some common symptoms of deficiencies.

Figure 16: ESSENTIAL B VITAMINS + DEFICIENCY SYMPTOMS

	8 Essential B Vitamins	Potential Deficiency Symptoms
B1	Thiamin (B1)	Beriberi, irregular heartbeat, edema
B2	Riboflavin (B2)	Cracked lips, inflammation, light sensitivity
B3	Niacin (B3)	Aggression, dermatitis, insomnia
B5	Pantothenic acid (B5)	Acne, tingling or numbness in skin
B6	Pyridoxal (B6)	Dermatitis, pink eye, neurological
B7	Biotin (B7)	May impair growth of infants
B9	Folate (folic acid) (B9)	May cause birth defects
B12	Cobalamin (B12)	Mania, psychosis

Vitamins B are water soluble. They must be consumed on a daily basis, as they are quickly flushed out of our system in our urine. As much as our bodies use and reuse the various components of essential fatty and essential amino acids, our bodies can take the essential vitamins B to create other vitamins B as needed.

But we must assure an adequate supply of the essentials, such as folate (B9, or folic acid) which our body uses to build our red blood cells.

The highest amounts of vitamins B are found in animal sources such as liver, tuna, and turkey. Whole grains, legumes, molasses, brewer's yeast, and nutritional yeast are other good sources.

Nutritional yeast contains a good amount of vitamins B. It has a slightly nutty flavor and can be sprinkled over popcorn, or added to sauces, stews, and soups for added flavor. There is also a fortified version of nutritional yeast which contains some amount of added vitamin B12. Vegetarians must be watchful to get enough of the essential vitamins B because some vegetation sources contain only limited amounts, especially for B12.

Stress is a factor that can deplete our vitamin B stores. Think of a time when you were driving in traffic and someone cut you off. Your mind recognized the imminent danger. Your body quickly responded by pressing on the brake in order to avoid a collision. As your body gets ready to respond automatically to the present danger, your foot quickly depresses the brake pedal. You may have noticed a "pins and needles" sensation throughout your body. That sensation is caused by your vitamin B stores being depleted from your cells so your brain can "think fast" and direct your body to respond appropriately to the present danger. After the stressful situation is resolved, you may find yourself feeling tired and drained from the experience. That's why we need to replenish our vitamin B stores daily. Our bodies tap into these stores regularly, and especially during any times of stress.

What is a shopper to do? It is important to note that just because the front label of a package claims that a product is "Whole Grain" does not mean that what is inside the package truly is. The words on the front label are most likely a marketing gimmick to mislead consumers.

We need to be "label readers." And if we can't pronounce any ingredient, we'd better be suspect, and look for an alternative option. Stuff like potato starch or tapioca starch are high glycemic ingredients popularly added to many products. They are a clear tip-off that you will be better left if you leave that product on the shelf at the store, rather than letting it rob you of your good health.

Whole grains also have a lot of fiber, phytochemicals, and potential anti-inflammatory and antioxidant properties, just the way nature intended. This is especially true when we compare whole grains to refined grains, which may be nearly devoid of any kind of nutrition that is recognized by our bodies.

Vani Hari, the "Food Babe" took social media by storm with her discoveries when she began publishing the results of some of her research on ingredient lists. Personally sickened by some of the unhealthy things added to processed foods, she began asking popular restaurants and food manufacturers questions about some of the ingredients that they were adding to their food products -- which they didn't want to answer. In many cases, the only way to get answers and effect change, was through designing public petitions. Her book *"The Food Babe Way"* details some of her work.[81]

Now we will turn our attention to some of the real whole grains that are available to include in our diets. Below is a little chart of some of the more popular whole grains in the USA. These whole grains are prepared by cooking in water, steaming, or even popping. Many of these "Whole Grain" foods are classified as seeds. But don't let the name fool you. The reality is that every whole grain really is a "seed." Each whole grain "seed" is capable of growing into an entire plant. Many of these "seeds" such as teff, chia, and quinoa are used as grains by many wise cooks in their practical kitchens.

Teff, for example, is a gluten-free "seed" grain ("grain" as defined by how we use it) that our bodies digest as other grains, like grains of whole wheat for example. The difference is that teff is a good option for those with a gluten intolerance. Teff can even be ground into a "flour" and used in baking, much the same as one might use whole wheat grains ground into flour. Or we can use the cooked, rinsed, and pureed legumes (beans, or pulses) to replace refined flour products as we talked about earlier.

An important note about all foods: Conventionally grown foods are likely genetically modified (and who knows exactly *what* has been done to any food during the genetic modification process). These conventionally grown foods (often referred to as "Frankenfoods) are typically sprayed with pesticides and/or herbicides which may be carcinogenic. And this applies to any and all conventionally grown foods of any kind. How can we tell if the foods are genetically modified and/or have been sprayed with these poisons? The problem is that genetically modified foods do not have to notify you that they are genetically modified or sprayed with poison. The burden is placed on organic foods, which bear the label "organic."

"Do you know they put glyphosate into our cereals?" an awestruck friend asked me the other day. It's not that glyphosate is directly added to our cereal, as in someone just added a scoop of glyphosate into each box of cereal as part of the manufacturing process for that product. Glyphosate is a product that conventional farmers use to kill the *weeds* that compete for the same nutrients as the genetically modified plant that produces the grains that are refined and processed into what finally *becomes* our cereal.

When a farmer spays crops with pesticides and herbicides, a full-body "hazmat" suit is needed for protection. The farmer does not inhale any excess vapor that may float into the air during the application. A gas mask is necessary for protection.

The plants in the field then absorb the toxic chemicals into themselves through the soil and water they use as they grow. They just can't help it. If these plants want to live, they must absorb water and nutrients from the soil. These chemicals become part of the plants as they mature on the farm. The majority of our corn, wheat and soy are likely contaminated as well. Then the plants are harvested and their grains removed. These grains are refined to produce the flours used as some of the ingredients in their recipes. The ingredients are all blended well and extruded to form the shapes of our cereals. Or our pastries, breads, donuts, muffins, cakes, etc. are also made with the refined flour that is created from the harvest of conventionally grown grains. Now, that is how glyphosate really gets into our cereal. It is innocently taken up by the plants during their growing process and simply becomes part of the grain produced by the mature plant. Refining the grains does not remove the glyphosate.

There is just no way to separate the glyphosate from the grain grown in a field where it is applied to keep down the weeds. So it just ends up as part of the cereal itself.

So back to the chart of whole grains. Most of the information included in the following chart is for cooked grains, but in a few cases we are talking about raw grains. And even though the subject is barely discussed when studying the basic nutritional macronutrients of our foods (like protein, carbohydrate, fiber, and fat), there is a HUGE difference in the quality of foods that are organic vs conventionally grown. That is, aside from the discussion of the glyphosate that is used in the farming of conventionally grown foods.

The chart lists each whole grain and whether it is cooked or raw. The typical serving size is shown in ounces, and the number of calories, amount of protein, carbs, fiber, and fat in that serving size are also shown. This chart lists our whole grains in alphabetical order:

Figure 17: WHOLE GRAINS MACRONUTRIENTS

GRAIN	OZ.	CAL	PROTEIN	CARBS	FIBER	FAT
Amaranth, cooked	5.29	153	6	28	3	2
Barley, pearled cooked	5.29	184	3	44	6	1
Buckwheat, cooked	5.29	138	5	30	4	1
Bulgur, cooked	5.29	124	5	28	7	0
Chia seeds, raw	1	138	5	12	10	9
Flax Seed, whole raw	1.5	100	3	6	6	4
Hemp seeds, whole	.5	90	4	1	1	7
Millet, cooked	5.29	178	5	36	2	2
Oats, steel cut, raw	1.34	142	4.75	26.65	3.8	2.4
Popcorn kernels, (2 Tbsp.)	1.16	121	3	23	5	2
Quinoa, boiled in water	5.29	180	7	32	4	3

NUTRIENT ESSENTIALS

GRAIN	OZ.	CAL	PROTEIN	CARBS	FIBER	FAT
Rice, Brown, steamed	5.29	225	5	46	3	3
Rye kernels, raw	1.5	54	2	12	2	0
Sweet corn, boiled, drained	5.29	144	5	31	4	2
Teff, cooked	5.29	152	6	30	4	1
Wheat Germ, raw	1.5	58	4	8	2	2
Wheat kernels, raw	1.5	37	2	6	2	0

82

FRUIT

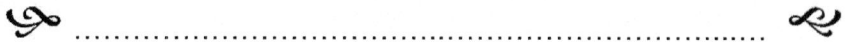

Fruits are botanically a part of the vegetable family, as well as are the nuts and seeds, legumes, and grains. After all, they are all vegetation, even though they are placed in their own section of the plate. MyPlate guidelines recommend that most adults consume between 1 ½ to 2 cups of fruit each day.

We will be looking at whole fruits, because whole fruits provide many more benefits than fruit juices. Even most 100% organic fruit juices lack fiber and other important nutrients that are vital components of the whole fruit. But first we will talk about those fruit juices, so we can set them aside and focus on the important micronutrients delivered to us as we eat our whole fruits.

To begin with, here is why that *fiber* we mentioned above is so important: Fiber creates bulk, and slows down the movement of food through our stomach and small intestine. Fiber keeps us feeling full longer and our blood sugar levels stable. When we eliminate that fiber by removing the juice of a fruit, we leave that juice open to be hastily digested and quickly converted into glucose. As that glucose quickly enters our bloodstream, the level of sugar in our blood goes up.

When our blood sugar goes up, our pancreas secretes insulin to bring it back down. That is the job of our pancreas. The insulin secreted by our pancreas takes that glucose and stores it as fat for our future use, like when we fast or face a famine. That is the job of insulin, and it does it very well.

But in our current culture, we don't need this storage. It may have come in handy for our ancestors, but in our culture today we have very little to no need for stored fat. We are not a hunter/gatherer society anymore. Instead of the forced fasting until we finally locate and secure our next meal, we have food available at all times. Today we are looking at about an eighty percent rate of *insulin resistance* in one degree or another. We just have too much insulin at work. And it is working to produce results that we do not want.

Knowing this, we are learning from our bodies. And we can work with our bodies to support and foster a more healthy physical being. What if we just gave our bodies a break from digestion, like our ancestors did?

What if we just left all types of nutrient tampered foods (AKA refined foods) out of our lives? How about if we no longer considered them among the choices we make to nourish our bodies? How about if we chose instead to select only the whole foods that are complete with all of their components like the complete profile of the essential fatty acids, amino acids, and vitamins B that they were born with? How about if we only gave our bodies foods that our bodies recognize and thus, through the wisdom of the ages, know just what to do with?

And if we have stored fat we'd like to burn off, why not just eat an early dinner, and then not eat again until breakfast the next day? This might equate to about an eighteen hour fast, allowing our body to focus its energy on cleaning up the excess debris of life, like errant mitochondria, free radicals, and other cellular waste in a process called *autophagy*. That is, rather than demanding that our body use energy to digest more food, like adding an evening snack that requires digestion.

The juices of all fruits have a high glycemic index (GI). They all convert quickly into sugar as they are digested. So now we will talk about real whole food. Our bodies need not the *caloric* density of juices, but the *nutrient* density of real foods in order to build health.

As you peal a fresh orange, grapefruit, or tangerine, you notice a while fibrous material just under the bright orange skin. This fibrous material is where the orange stores its antioxidant bioflavonoids. Bioflavonoids, also known as flavonoids, protect our cells against free radical damage. Free radicals can damage our healthy cells. This damage is a form of oxidative stress. Antioxidants may even slow, or prevent aging, cancer, allergies, and other diseases. There are 4,000 to 6,000 known bioflavonoids. They can help our bodies absorb and use vitamin C.

Good sources of bioflavonoids include almonds, apples, bananas, cherries, cranberries, citrus fruits, onions, quinoa, turnip greens, watermelon, and green and black tea.

An apple stores most of its nutrition just under its skin. As you bite into one, you notice that this is also the most flavorful part of the apple. Apples are a great source of pectin, a type of gelatinous fiber that lowers cholesterol. And scientific research points to some health building benefits when we eat certain fruits. For instance, those fruits with deep colors are found especially helpful.

Those deep colors are caused by one particular bioflavonoid, *anthocyanin.* While the Food and Drug Administration (FDA) may not currently recommend anthocyanin consumption for health benefits, the National Institutes of Health is one step ahead of the FDA.

On August 15, 2018 the *National Institutes of Health* presented their findings in a research review published by the National

Institute of Diabetes and Digestive and Kidney Disease that states "consumption of anthocyanin-rich foods, particularly blueberries and apples/pears, was associated with lower risk of type 2 diabetes (72)."[83] [84]

Anthocyanins are powerful anti-oxidants and anti-inflammatory micronutrients. Oxidation and inflammation are at the heart of most non-communicable diseases like cancer, heart disease, and type 2 diabetes. Blueberries, apples, and pears all have a low glycemic index (GI).

Fruits also provide vitamin C, essential to healing and maintaining healthy teeth and gums. Many fruits provide potassium, which can lower blood pressure. A diet that includes plenty of fruits and vegetables may also reduce our risk for heart attack and stroke.

Focusing on whole fruits like blueberries, apples, and pears that bring to your body the advantageous properties of anthocyanins can be a very good choice, indeed. This is particularly so for individuals with concerns of insulin resistance, prediabetes, or type 2 diabetes. Keep in mind, though, that some fruits may be much higher in carbohydrate content as well as glycemic index than other sources of vegetation.

Here is a little chart that shows you the typical serving sizes in ounces, the number of calories, protein, carbohydrate, fiber and fat in about 45 of our most popular fruits. The fruits are listed here in alphabetical order, so you can quickly locate your favorites and see how they compare. Most serving sizes are about 4 ¼ ounce (120 g.).:

Figure 18: FRUITS MACRONUTRIENTS

FRUIT	OZ.	CAL	PROTEIN	CARBS	FIBER	FAT
Apple	4.23	63	0.3	16	3	0.2
Apricot	4.23	56	1.7	13	2	0.4

FRUIT

FRUIT	OZ.	CAL	PROTEIN	CARBS	FIBER	FAT
Avocado	4.23	192	2.4	11	8	17
Banana, average	4.23	107	1.3	25	3	0.4
Boysenberries	4.23	105	1.2	14	6	0.1
Blackberries	4.23	52	1.7	12	4	0.6
Blueberries	4.23	69	0.9	17	3	0.4
Cantaloupe	4.23	40	1	10	1	0.2
Cherries, red	4.23	60	1.2	14	2	0.4
Cranberries	4.23	55	0.5	14	6	1.5
Dates	2.12	166	1.09	43	5	0.09
Figs	0.99	70	0.92	8	1	0.26
Grapefruit	4.23	51	0.9	8	2	0.2
Grapes, Black	4.23	78	0.86	21	1	0.86
Guava	4.23	83	3.1	17	6	1.1
Honeydew	4.23	43	0.6	11	1	0.2
Kiwi	4.23	73	1.4	18	4	0.7
Lychee	4.23	75	1.2	20	2	0
Mandarin	4.23	64	1	16	2	0.37
Mango	4.23	72	1	18	2	0.5
Mulberries	4.23	48	1.6	12	2	0.8
Oranges	4.23	56	1.1	11	3	0.1
Papaya	4.23	52	0.56	13	2	0.31
Passionfruit	4.23	113	2.7	28	12	0.7
Peach, fresh	4.23	47	1.1	12	2	0.3
Peaches, canned in light syrup	4.23	65	0.54	17	2	0.04
Pear, fresh	4.23	69	0.4	18	4	0.1
Pear, canned in pear juice	4.23	58	0	11	4	0
Persimmon	4.23	153	1	41	4	0.5
Pineapple	4.23	60	0.6	16	2	0.1
Plantain	4.23	146	1.5	38	3	0.5
Plum	4.23	55	0.84	13	2	0.34
Pomegranate	4.23	99	2.1	23	9	1.4
Prunes, pitted	2.12	150	1.5	33	4	0
Raisins	2.12	178	1.51	47	2	0.32
Raspberries	4.23	63	1.5	15	8	0.8
Rhubarb	4.23	26	1.1	5	2	0.2
Rose hips	0.99	45	.45	11	7	0.10

FRUIT	OZ.	CAL	PROTEIN	CARBS	FIBER	FAT
Soursop	4.23	79	1	20	4	0.4
Strawberries	4.23	40	1	3	2	0
Tangerine	4.23	64	1	16	2	0.4
Tomato	4.23	22	1.06	4.67	1.4	0.24
Watermelon	4.23	36	0.7	10	1	0.2

85

In the last three chapters, we have looked at how we can fulfill our bodies' nutrient essentials. We have also considered the recommended food group allotments for a well-rounded diet according to MyPlate guidelines.

We have seen the macronutrients of our foods placed into their food groups. This allowed us to compare the foods, one against another in each group for their calories, protein, carbohydrate, fiber and fat content in alphabetical order. Hopefully, this made it easier to compare the macronutrients they contain to the others in their particular food group. And with any luck at all, you might have found some new ideas along the way.

Now we're going to look at all of these foods in a different way that may give us a new perspective.

PERSPECTIVES

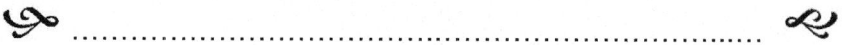

T his chapter of the book holds some very special charts. If you are evaluating your meal patterns, these next charts may be useful to you.

- The first chart organizes foods by the number of calories they contain in a typical serving. Foods with the least number of calories per serving are at the top of the chart. If you are looking to add lower calorie foods, you might focus on the top third of the foods in this chart. Foods containing the greatest number of calories are at the bottom of the chart.

- The second chart organizes foods by the amount of protein they contain in a typical serving. Foods containing the greatest amount of protein are at the top of the chart. If you are looking to add some high protein foods to your meal plan, you might focus on the top third of the foods in this chart. Foods that contain the least amount of protein are at the bottom of the chart.

- The third chart shows the amount of carbohydrate in a typical serving. Foods with the least amount of carbohydrate are at the top of the chart. If you are looking for low carbohydrate foods, you might focus on the top third of the foods in this chart. Foods with the greatest amount of carbohydrate are at the bottom of the chart.

- The forth chart shows the amount fiber (fibre) in a typical serving. Foods with the greatest amount of fiber are at the top of the chart. If you are looking to increase your intake of fiber, you might focus on the foods at the top third of the chart. Foods with the least amount of fiber are at the bottom of the chart.

- The fifth chart shows the amount of fat in a typical serving. Foods with the least amount of fat are at the top of the chart. If you want to reduce the amount of fat in your diet, you might focus on the foods listed in the top third of the chart. Foods with the greatest amount of fat are at the bottom of the chart.

CALORIES FROM LOW TO HIGH

Now we're going to look at all of our vegetation sourced foods by the number of calories they contain. Calories are important as they represent the amount of energy we consume. If you are looking for calorie counts, I hope this next chart is helpful to you. The chart shows you the amount of calories in a typical serving of these foods. So if you are looking to add some low calorie choices to your meal plan, you will find the foods with the least number of calories right at the top of this chart. The number of calories increase all the way to the end of the chart, where those foods with the greatest number of calories are listed. You might find some interesting selections here among the first few pages:

Figure 19: CALORIES FROM LOW TO HIGH

FOOD	OZ.	CAL
Radish	1.06	5
Watercress	4.23	13
Bok Choy	4.23	17
Celery	4.23	17
Cucumber	4.23	18
Asparagus	4.23	20
Green Leaf Lettuce	5.29	22
Bell pepper	4.23	22
Tomato	4.23	22

FOOD	OZ.	CAL
Ginger root	0.99	22
Tomato	4.23	22
Swiss chard	4.23	23
Artichoke	4.23	23
Zucchini	4.23	25
Mushrooms, white	4.23	26
Beet greens	4.23	26
Rhubarb	4.23	26
Radicchio	4.23	28
Arugula	4.23	30
Wheatgrass* powder, organic, dry	.33	30
Cauliflower	4.23	30
Cabbage	4.23	30
Eggplant	4.23	30
Mustard greens	4.23	32
Kohlrabi	4.23	32
Parsnips	2.82	32
Spinach	5.29	34
Watermelon	4.23	36
Green beans	4.23	37
Wheat kernels, raw	1.5	37
Collard greens	4.23	38
Tomatillo	4.23	38
Okra	4.23	40
Cantaloupe	4.23	40
Strawberries	4.23	40
Broccoli	4.23	41
Kale	4.23	42
Garlic	0.99	42
Honeydew	4.23	43
Rose hips	0.99	45
Jicama	4.23	46
Peach, fresh	4.23	47
Mulberries	4.23	48
Onion	4.23	48
Carrots	4.23	49
Nopal (prickly pear cactus)	4.23	49

NUTRIENT ESSENTIALS

FOOD	OZ.	CAL
Grapefruit	4.23	51
Blackberries	4.23	52
Papaya	4.23	52
Dandelion greens	4.23	54
Rye kernels, raw	1.5	54
Plum	4.23	55
Cranberries	4.23	55
Grape leaves	2.12	56
Apricot	4.23	56
Oranges	4.23	56
Wheat Germ	1.5	58
Pear, canned in pear juice	4.23	58
Cherries, red	4.23	60
Pineapple	4.23	60
Raspberries	4.23	63
Apple	4.23	63
Mandarin	4.23	64
Tangerine	4.23	64
Green Peas	2.82	65
Peaches, canned in light syrup	4.23	65
Blueberries	4.23	69
Pear, fresh	4.23	69
Figs	0.99	70
Mango	4.23	72
Leek	4.23	73
Kiwi	4.23	73
Lychee	4.23	75
Grapes, Black	4.23	78
Soursop	4.23	79
Guava	4.23	83
Turmeric powder	.99	87
Potato, baked russet	5.29	89
Pomegranate	4.23	99
Flax Seed, whole raw	1.5	100
Boysenberries	4.23	105
Banana, average	4.23	107
Passionfruit	4.23	113
Popcorn kernels, (2 Tbsp.)	1.16	121
Bulgur, cooked	5.29	124

FOOD	OZ.	CAL
Potato, sweet, baked	5.29	135
Fava/broad beans	5.29	138
Buckwheat, cooked	5.29	138
Chia seeds, raw	1	138
Oats, steel cut, raw	1.34	142
Sweet corn, boiled, drained	5.29	144
Plantain	4.23	146
Prunes, pitted	2.12	150
Teff, cooked	5.29	152
Amaranth, cooked	5.29	153
Persimmon	4.23	153
Garbanzo/Chickpeas, boiled	5.29	165
Dates	2.12	166
Olives, plain	4.23	168
Soybean sprouts	5.29	171
Tofu	5.29	174
Potato, yam, average	5.29	174
Soybeans (edamame)	5.29	177
Millet, cooked	5.29	178
Raisins	2.12	178
Quinoa, boiled in water	5.29	180
Lentils, boiled	5.29	182
Lima beans, boiled	5.29	184
Pinto beans	5.29	184
Barley, pearled cooked	5.29	184
Avocado	4.23	192
Black beans, boiled	5.29	198
Haricot / Navy beans, boiled	5.29	207
Kidney beans, boiled	5.29	210
Split peas	5.29	212
Rice, Brown, steamed	5.29	225
Pepitas	1.76	266
Pistachios	1.76	280
Cashews	1.76	281
Peanuts	1.76	284
Sunflower seeds	1.76	284
Sesame seeds	1.76	286
Almonds	1.76	298
Filberts/Hazelnuts	1.76	314

FOOD	OZ.	CAL
Pumpkin seeds	1.76	320
Walnuts	1.76	334
Pecans	1.76	340
Macadamia	1.76	359

86

Now we're going to look at how we might expand our protein options by looking at our food sources for protein from a different perspective. This will let us see how all of these individual foods stack up against each other as we keep an eye on eating the recommended 150 -160 g. of protein each day.

PROTEIN FROM HIGH TO LOW

The following chart is comprised of all the charts of foods we have looked at alphabetically in their different food groups, such as vegetables, nuts and seeds, legumes, whole grains, and fruits. These are all vegetation type foods. They grow in your yard, on a farm, or even in containers. The plants that produce these treasures get their nourishment from the dirt and the decomposition of organic materials that are in the dirt. That puts them low on the food chain, just like the algae or krill we talked about in the fatty acid chapter. All of these foods provide a certain amount of protein when eaten in typical serving sizes.

In this chart, again, foods are presented in their typical serving sizes. The typical serving size and the amount of protein in each serving are listed. But the difference is that all of these foods are organized by the *amount* of *protein* they contain. Foods with the most protein per serving are at the top of this chart. Foods with the least amount of protein are at the bottom of the chart. This might be helpful to you if your goal is to add more protein to your meal plans. In this case, you might start with some of the foods toward the top of this chart, since they have the most protein:

Figure 20: PROTEIN FROM HIGH TO LOW

FOOD	OZ.	PROTEIN
Soybeans (edamame)	5.29	19
Split peas	5.29	19
Pumpkin seeds	1.76	18
Pepitas	1.76	15
Tofu	5.29	13
Black beans, boiled	5.29	13
Peanuts	1.76	13
Lentils, boiled	5.29	12
Sunflower seeds	1.76	12
Garbanzo/Chickpeas, boiled	5.29	11
Haricot / Navy beans, boiled	5.29	11
Kidney beans, boiled	5.29	11
Almonds	1.76	11
Soybean sprouts	5.29	10
Lima beans, boiled	5.29	10
Pinto beans	5.29	10
Pistachios	1.76	10
Cashews	1.76	10
Sesame seeds	1.76	9
Fava/broad beans	5.29	8
Walnuts	1.76	8
Quinoa, boiled in water	5.29	7
Filberts/Hazelnuts	1.76	7
Teff, cooked	5.29	6
Amaranth, cooked	5.29	6
Bulgur, cooked	5.29	5
Buckwheat, cooked	5.29	5
Chia seeds, raw	1	5
Sweet corn, boiled, drained	5.29	5
Millet, cooked	5.29	5
Rice, Brown, steamed	5.29	5
Pecans	1.76	5
Oats, steel cut, raw	1.34	4.75
Spinach	5.29	4.29
Wheat Germ	1.5	4
Green Peas	2.82	4

NUTRIENT ESSENTIALS

FOOD	OZ.	PROTEIN
Macadamia	1.76	4
Collard greens	4.23	3.78
Kale	4.23	3.65
Mushrooms, white	4.23	3.64
Mustard greens	4.23	3.6
Broccoli	4.23	3.38
Dandelion greens	4.23	3.38
Grape leaves	2.12	3.36
Arugula	4.23	3.24
Guava	4.23	3.1
Swiss chard	4.23	3
Watercress	4.23	3
Zucchini	4.23	3
Wheatgrass* powder, organic, dry	.33	3
Potato, baked russet	5.29	3
Flax Seed, whole raw	1.5	3
Popcorn kernels, (2 Tbsp.)	1.16	3
Potato, sweet, baked	5.29	3
Barley, pearled cooked	5.29	3
Turmeric powder	.99	2.87
Asparagus	4.23	2.75
Beet greens	4.23	2.75
Passionfruit	4.23	2.7
Artichoke	4.23	2.5
Okra	4.23	2.41
Cauliflower	4.23	2.4
Avocado	4.23	2.4
Green beans	4.23	2.29
Kohlrabi	4.23	2.13
Pomegranate	4.23	2.1
Green Leaf Lettuce	5.29	2
Wheat kernels, raw	1.5	2
Garlic	0.99	2
Rye kernels, raw	1.5	2
Potato, yam, average	5.29	2
Leek	4.23	1.88
Radicchio	4.23	1.72
Blackberries	4.23	1.7

FOOD	OZ.	PROTEIN
Apricot	4.23	1.7
Cabbage	4.23	1.6
Mulberries	4.23	1.6
Raisins	2.12	1.51
Raspberries	4.23	1.5
Plantain	4.23	1.5
Prunes, pitted	2.12	1.5
Bok Choy	4.23	1.48
Bell pepper	4.23	1.48
Kiwi	4.23	1.4
Onion	4.23	1.38
Banana, average	4.23	1.3
Eggplant	4.23	1.22
Cherries, red	4.23	1.2
Lychee	4.23	1.2
Boysenberries	4.23	1.2
Rhubarb	4.23	1.1
Peach, fresh	4.23	1.1
Oranges	4.23	1.1
Dates	2.12	1.09
Tomato	4.23	1.06
Ginger root	0.99	1
Tomato	4.23	1
Parsnips	2.82	1
Tomatillo	4.23	1
Cantaloupe	4.23	1
Strawberries	4.23	1
Carrots	4.23	1
Nopal (prickly pear cactus)	4.23	1
Mandarin	4.23	1
Tangerine	4.23	1
Mango	4.23	1
Soursop	4.23	1
Persimmon	4.23	1
Figs	0.99	0.92
Grapefruit	4.23	0.9
Blueberries	4.23	0.9
Celery	4.23	0.86

FOOD	OZ.	PROTEIN
Jicama	4.23	0.86
Grapes, Black	4.23	0.86
Plum	4.23	0.84
Cucumber	4.23	0.81
Watermelon	4.23	0.7
Honeydew	4.23	0.6
Pineapple	4.23	0.6
Papaya	4.23	0.56
Peaches, canned in light syrup	4.23	0.54
Cranberries	4.23	0.5
Rose hips	0.99	.45
Pear, fresh	4.23	0.4
Apple	4.23	0.3
Radish	1.06	.20

87

We can see that all vegetation does provide some protein.
Soybeans and split peas offer 19 g. per serving, while pumpkin
seeds and pepitas come in at 18 and 15 g. respectively. But you
would have to eat over seven servings of soybeans or split peas a
day to meet the required 150 g. of protein. So if you are
considering a strict vegetarian diet, you may want to do a bit of
research to be sure you are able to meet your needs for protein.
You may want to study the practice of combining certain different
foods at each meal in order to increase the amount of protein that
each meal delivers.

CARBOHYDRATES FROM LOW TO HIGH

This chart shows you the number of carbohydrates there are in
vegetarian food sources. If you are counting your carbs, you may
find this chart helpful. It lists carbohydrate in these vegetarian
foods from low to high. This might make it useful in locating low
carb food choices. Foods with the least amount of carbs are at the
top of the chart:

Figure 21: CARBOHYDRATES FROM LOW TO HIGH

FOOD	OZ.	CARBS
Radish	1.06	1
Watercress	4.23	2
Strawberries	4.23	3
Spinach	5.29	4
Mushrooms, white	4.23	4
Arugula	4.23	4
Swiss chard	4.23	4
Zucchini	4.23	4
Green Leaf Lettuce	5.29	4
Celery	4.23	4
Cucumber	4.23	4
Tomato	4.23	4.67
Pepitas	1.76	5
Asparagus	4.23	5
Rhubarb	4.23	5
Ginger root	0.99	5
Tomato	4.23	5
Radicchio	4.23	5.38
Pumpkin seeds	1.76	6
Collard greens	4.23	6
Wheatgrass* powder, organic, dry	.33	6
Flax Seed, whole raw	1.5	6
Cauliflower	4.23	6
Wheat kernels, raw	1.5	6
Walnuts	1.76	7
Pecans	1.76	7
Macadamia	1.76	7
Mustard greens	4.23	7
Kohlrabi	4.23	7
Cabbage	4.23	7
Bok Choy	4.23	7
Eggplant	4.23	7
Tomatillo	4.23	7
Olives, plain	4.23	7
Peanuts	1.76	8
Filberts/Hazelnuts	1.76	8

NUTRIENT ESSENTIALS

FOOD	OZ.	CARBS
Wheat Germ	1.5	8
Broccoli	4.23	8
Okra	4.23	8
Green beans	4.23	8
Figs	0.99	8
Grapefruit	4.23	8
Garlic	0.99	9
Sunflower seeds	1.76	10
Grape leaves	2.12	10
Cantaloupe	4.23	10
Watermelon	4.23	10
Almonds	1.76	11
Kale	4.23	11
Dandelion greens	4.23	11
Avocado	4.23	11
Bell pepper	4.23	11
Onion	4.23	11
Oranges	4.23	11
Nopal (prickly pear cactus)	4.23	11
Jicama	4.23	11
Honeydew	4.23	11
Rose hips	0.99	11
Pear, canned in pear juice	4.23	11
Sesame seeds	1.76	12
Chia seeds, raw	1	12
Green Peas	2.82	12
Beet greens	4.23	12
Rye kernels, raw	1.5	12
Blackberries	4.23	12
Mulberries	4.23	12
Peach, fresh	4.23	12
Carrots	4.23	12
Artichoke	4.23	13
Apricot	4.23	13
Plum	4.23	13
Papaya	4.23	13
Soybeans (edamame)	5.29	14
Pistachios	1.76	14
Cashews	1.76	14

FOOD	OZ.	CARBS
Cherries, red	4.23	14
Boysenberries	4.23	14
Parsnips	2.82	14
Cranberries	4.23	14
Raspberries	4.23	15
Mandarin	4.23	16
Tangerine	4.23	16
Pineapple	4.23	16
Apple	4.23	16
Split peas	5.29	17
Guava	4.23	17
Leek	4.23	17
Blueberries	4.23	17
Peaches, canned in light syrup	4.23	17
Kiwi	4.23	18
Mango	4.23	18
Pear, fresh	4.23	18
Turmeric powder	.99	19
Lychee	4.23	20
Soursop	4.23	20
Grapes, Black	4.23	21
Popcorn kernels, (2 Tbsp.)	1.16	23
Pomegranate	4.23	23
Fava/broad beans	5.29	24
Banana, average	4.23	25
Potato, baked russet	5.29	26
Oats, steel cut, raw	1.34	26.65
Amaranth, cooked	5.29	28
Bulgur, cooked	5.29	28
Passionfruit	4.23	28
Garbanzo/Chickpeas, boiled	5.29	29
Soybean sprouts	5.29	30
Teff, cooked	5.29	30
Buckwheat, cooked	5.29	30
Tofu	5.29	31
Lentils, boiled	5.29	31
Sweet corn, boiled, drained	5.29	31
Potato, sweet, baked	5.29	31
Quinoa, boiled in water	5.29	32

FOOD	OZ.	CARBS
Prunes, pitted	2.12	33
Haricot / Navy beans, boiled	5.29	34
Black beans, boiled	5.29	35
Lima beans, boiled	5.29	35
Pinto beans	5.29	35
Millet, cooked	5.29	36
Plantain	4.23	38
Kidney beans, boiled	5.29	39
Persimmon	4.23	41
Potato, yam, average	5.29	42
Dates	2.12	43
Barley, pearled cooked	5.29	44
Rice, Brown, steamed	5.29	46
Raisins	2.12	47

88

FIBER FROM HIGH TO LOW

Fiber is a component of many of our foods. Dietary fibers (fibre) are mainly hygroscopic (soak up water) complex carbohydrates that come from plant cell walls, like cellulose, hemicellulose, and pectin. Be sure to drink enough water so that fiber can do its job. While our recommended daily allowance of fiber is for about 30 – 50 grams, many of us get only about 5 grams for one reason or another. This chart might be helpful to you because foods with the most fiber are at the top of the chart, foods with the least amount of fiber are at the bottom of this chart:

Figure 22: FIBER FROM HIGH TO LOW

FOOD	OZ.	FIBER
Kidney beans, boiled	5.29	15
Tofu	5.29	13
Black beans, boiled	5.29	13
Passionfruit	4.23	12
Chia seeds, raw	1	10
Lentils, boiled	5.29	9
Haricot / Navy beans, boiled	5.29	9

FOOD	OZ.	FIBER
Mustard greens	4.23	9
Pomegranate	4.23	9
Garbanzo/Chickpeas, boiled	5.29	8
Soybean sprouts	5.29	8
Lima beans, boiled	5.29	8
Pinto beans	5.29	8
Avocado	4.23	8
Raspberries	4.23	8
Bulgur, cooked	5.29	7
Grape leaves	2.12	7
Rose hips	0.99	7
Split peas	5.29	6
Almonds	1.76	6
Sesame seeds	1.76	6
Guava	4.23	6
Flax Seed, whole raw	1.5	6
Barley, pearled cooked	5.29	6
Turmeric powder	.99	6
Artichoke	4.23	6
Potato, yam, average	5.29	6
Boysenberries	4.23	6
Jicama	4.23	6
Cranberries	4.23	6
Sunflower seeds	1.76	5
Pistachios	1.76	5
Fava/broad beans	5.29	5
Filberts/Hazelnuts	1.76	5
Pecans	1.76	5
Green Peas	2.82	5
Collard greens	4.23	5
Popcorn kernels, (2 Tbsp.)	1.16	5
Potato, sweet, baked	5.29	5
Dates	2.12	5
Soybeans (edamame)	5.29	4
Pumpkin seeds	1.76	4
Peanuts	1.76	4
Walnuts	1.76	4
Quinoa, boiled in water	5.29	4
Teff, cooked	5.29	4

NUTRIENT ESSENTIALS

FOOD	OZ.	FIBER
Buckwheat, cooked	5.29	4
Sweet corn, boiled, drained	5.29	4
Macadamia	1.76	4
Dandelion greens	4.23	4
Okra	4.23	4
Green beans	4.23	4
Kohlrabi	4.23	4
Blackberries	4.23	4
Prunes, pitted	2.12	4
Kiwi	4.23	4
Eggplant	4.23	4
Parsnips	2.82	4
Nopal (prickly pear cactus)	4.23	4
Soursop	4.23	4
Persimmon	4.23	4
Pear, fresh	4.23	4
Pear, canned in pear juice	4.23	4
Olives, plain	4.23	4
Oats, steel cut, raw	1.34	3.8
Pepitas	1.76	3
Amaranth, cooked	5.29	3
Rice, Brown, steamed	5.29	3
Spinach	5.29	3
Broccoli	4.23	3
Wheatgrass* powder, organic, dry	.33	3
Asparagus	4.23	3
Beet greens	4.23	3
Cabbage	4.23	3
Plantain	4.23	3
Banana, average	4.23	3
Oranges	4.23	3
Carrots	4.23	3
Blueberries	4.23	3
Apple	4.23	3
Potato, baked russet	5.29	2.1
Cashews	1.76	2
Millet, cooked	5.29	2
Wheat Germ	1.5	2
Kale	4.23	2

FOOD	OZ.	FIBER
Arugula	4.23	2
Swiss chard	4.23	2
Cauliflower	4.23	2
Green Leaf Lettuce	5.29	2
Wheat kernels, raw	1.5	2
Rye kernels, raw	1.5	2
Leek	4.23	2
Apricot	4.23	2
Mulberries	4.23	2
Raisins	2.12	2
Bell pepper	4.23	2
Onion	4.23	2
Cherries, red	4.23	2
Lychee	4.23	2
Rhubarb	4.23	2
Peach, fresh	4.23	2
Tomatillo	4.23	2
Strawberries	4.23	2
Mandarin	4.23	2
Tangerine	4.23	2
Mango	4.23	2
Grapefruit	4.23	2
Celery	4.23	2
Plum	4.23	2
Pineapple	4.23	2
Papaya	4.23	2
Peaches, canned in light syrup	4.23	2
Tomato	4.23	1.4
Mushrooms, white	4.23	1
Watercress	4.23	1
Zucchini	4.23	1
Garlic	0.99	1
Radicchio	4.23	1
Bok Choy	4.23	1
Ginger root	0.99	1
Tomato	4.23	1
Cantaloupe	4.23	1
Figs	0.99	1

NUTRIENT ESSENTIALS

FOOD	OZ.	FIBER
Grapes, Black	4.23	1
Cucumber	4.23	1
Watermelon	4.23	1
Honeydew	4.23	1
Radish	1.06	1

89

FAT FROM LOW TO HIGH

Here is another interesting chart you might find helpful. It lists the amount of fats in our vegetarian food sources. Foods that contain the least amount of fats are at the top of the chart; foods with the greatest amount of fats are at the bottom of the chart:

Figure 23: FATS FROM LOW TO HIGH

FOOD	OZ.	FAT
Radish	1.06	.03
Peaches, canned in light syrup	4.23	.04
Parsnips	2.82	.08
Dates	2.12	.09
Boysenberries	4.23	0.1
Oranges	4.23	0.1
Pineapple	4.23	0.1
Rose hips	0.99	.10
Pear, fresh	4.23	0.1
Jicama	4.23	.11
Kohlrabi	4.23	.12
Onion	4.23	.12
Cucumber	4.23	.13
Watercress	4.23	0.2
Rhubarb	4.23	0.2
Cantaloupe	4.23	0.2
Grapefruit	4.23	0.2
Celery	4.23	0.2
Watermelon	4.23	0.2
Honeydew	4.23	0.2
Apple	4.23	0.2
Ginger root	0.99	.21
Green Leaf Lettuce	5.29	.22
Eggplant	4.23	.22
Potato, sweet, baked	5.29	.23
Okra	4.23	.23
Potato, yam, average	5.29	.23
Swiss chard	4.23	.24
Tomato	4.23	.24
Tomato	4.23	.24

NUTRIENT ESSENTIALS

FOOD	OZ.	FAT
Green beans	4.23	.26
Figs	0.99	.26
Carrots	4.23	.29
Radicchio	4.23	.30
Peach, fresh	4.23	0.3
Papaya	4.23	.31
Green Peas	2.82	.32
Raisins	2.12	.32
Cauliflower	4.23	.34
Plum	4.23	.34
Leek	4.23	.36
Mandarin	4.23	.37
Apricot	4.23	0.4
Banana, average	4.23	0.4
Cherries, red	4.23	0.4
Tangerine	4.23	0.4
Soursop	4.23	0.4
Blueberries	4.23	0.4
Mushrooms, white	4.23	.41
Zucchini	4.23	.48
Mustard greens	4.23	.5
Plantain	4.23	0.5
Mango	4.23	0.5
Persimmon	4.23	0.5
Spinach	5.29	.58
Garlic	0.99	0.6
Blackberries	4.23	0.6
Nopal (prickly pear cactus)	4.23	.61
Passionfruit	4.23	.7
Kiwi	4.23	0.7
Collard greens	4.23	.73
Mulberries	4.23	0.8
Raspberries	4.23	0.8
Dandelion greens	4.23	.84
Grapes, Black	4.23	.86
Turmeric powder	.99	.91
Black beans, boiled	5.29	1
Lentils, boiled	5.29	1
Garbanzo/Chickpeas, boiled	5.29	1

PERSPECTIVES: FAT FROM LOW TO HIGH

FOOD	OZ.	FAT
Kidney beans, boiled	5.29	1
Soybean sprouts	5.29	1
Fava/broad beans	5.29	1
Teff, cooked	5.29	1
Buckwheat, cooked	5.29	1
Arugula	4.23	1
Barley, pearled cooked	5.29	1
Guava	4.23	1.1
Tomatillo	4.23	1.2
Grape leaves	2.12	1.3
Pomegranate	4.23	1.4
Cranberries	4.23	1.5
Kale	4.23	1.8
Amaranth, cooked	5.29	2
Sweet corn, boiled, drained	5.29	2
Millet, cooked	5.29	2
Wheat Germ	1.5	2
Popcorn kernels, (2 Tbsp.)	1.16	2
Oats, steel cut, raw	1.34	2.4
Quinoa, boiled in water	5.29	3
Rice, Brown, steamed	5.29	3
Flax Seed, whole raw	1.5	4
Filberts/Hazelnuts	1.76	4.8
Pistachios	1.76	5
Haricot / Navy beans, boiled	5.29	9
Chia seeds, raw	1	9
Split peas	5.29	10
Soybeans (edamame)	5.29	11
Tofu	5.29	13
Avocado	4.23	17
Olives, plain	4.23	18
Cashews	1.76	22
Pepitas	1.76	23
Peanuts	1.76	25
Sunflower seeds	1.76	25
Almonds	1.76	25
Sesame seeds	1.76	25
Pumpkin seeds	1.76	28
Walnuts	1.76	33

NUTRIENT ESSENTIALS

FOOD	OZ.	FAT
Pecans	1.76	36
Macadamia	1.76	38

90

DAIRY & ALTERNATIVES

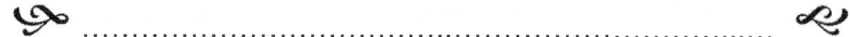

Dairy is the most commonly promoted vehicle for our calcium intake, and the guidance given for MyPlate is no exception. Our bodies need calcium to build and rebuild strong bones, teeth, and so much more. And beginning at the age of 9 years, the recommendation is that we all consume the equivalent of 3 glasses of cow's milk each day. (Nowhere else in nature does any animal consume the milk of another species past weaning from their Mother's breast.) And we have an abundance of cow's milk in this country.

But the fact is that over 60% of adults have a problem digesting *any* kind of dairy products. So what about us? What about our needs? While we could substitute a slice of some cheeses or a cup of yogurt to replace milk for our recommended dairy requirement, most of us have a problem digesting any of these dairy products at all.

Speaking of facts, based on statistics, the ability to digest milk past childhood is what is really unusual. That's because being able to digest milk past childhood is so strange that scientists say we shouldn't really call lactose intolerance a "disease," because considering it a disease makes it seem like this is *abnormal*. But in normal humans, the enzyme produced by our bodies to digest milk, called lactase, is no longer produced by our small intestines after we reach about two to five years of age. That equates to about the time most of us are weaned from our Mother's breasts, according to the schedule of nature.

What happens to us instead when our bodies no longer produce the enzyme lactase, is that the undigested milk sugars – called lactose -- end up in our colon, where they begin to ferment, producing gas that can cause cramping, bloating, nausea, flatulence and diarrhea.

Less than 40% of adults worldwide maintain the ability to digest lactose past childhood.[91] And as many as 75% of our African and Native Americans and 90% of our Asian Americans have what is called "lactose intolerance." That's according to our National Institute of Diabetes and Digestive and Kidney Diseases (NIDDK.)

Symptoms of *lactose intolerance* include bloating, diarrhea, gas, nausea, and stomach cramps. And some may even vomit right after consuming lactose. The less violent symptoms usually kick in half an hour to two hours after eating foods that contain lactose. The vomiting may happen almost immediately in highly sensitive individuals – and maybe they are better off -- because they get to skip the gastrointestinal problems created when lactose gets to their colon.

If you find that you are lactose intolerant, be certain to read ingredient labels – and especially on all of the following foods that may contain added lactose:

Figure 24: LACTOSE CONTAINING FOODS

- breads and baked goods of any kind, fresh, frozen, or box mixes
- candies, chips, and other snack foods
- cereals in boxes or bags
- frozen dinners
- instant breakfast drinks, protein drinks, and soup mixes
- Instant potatoes, and instant potato products

- lunch meats (that are not kosher)
- margarines of any kind
- Prepared mixes for cakes, cookies, biscuits, pancakes and waffles, etc.
- salad dressings, in jars or prepared packaged salad dressing mixes

As you read your ingredient labels carefully, be aware that there are also some inventive names that are used for many lactose-based ingredients. You'll also want to be on the lookout for any of these. Manufacturers may list lactose-based ingredients used in their recipes by some of these names:

Figure 25: OTHER NAMES FOR LACTOSE

- artificial and natural butter flavor
- butter
- caramel flavor or coloring, sometimes
- caseinate, of any kind (i.e. iron or potassium, etc.)
- cheese
- condensed milk
- cream
- curds
- demineralized whey
- dried milk
- enriched flour, sometimes
- evaporated milk
- Formaige frais
- ghee
- high protein flour, sometimes
- hydrolysates
- hydrolyzed vegetable protein
- lacalbumin
- lactose-free milk
- lactate solids

- lactulose
- lactogloblin
- lactobumin
- lactobum phosphate
- lactoferrin
- margarine
- milk
- milk derivative
- milk solids
- nougat
- powdered milk
- quark
- recaldent
- rennet
- sodium caseinate
- whey
- yogurt

The above ingredients are all dairy-based and able to cause the uncomfortable effects we talked about earlier.

There are lactase supplements available that may reduce or even eliminate some of the symptoms of lactose intolerance. These are available over the counter.

Be aware that this supplement must be taken BEFORE you consume any lactose at all in order to do their work. They are not effective if you take them AFTER you consume a dairy product of any kind and begin to experience any symptoms.

As we have seen, more than half of us have trouble digesting any kind of dairy products. In fact, current estimates point out that 60% of us suffer with symptoms due to our *normal* intolerance to lactose. The symptoms present themselves whenever we consume dairy products of any kind. And I know the list is long for ingredients that may be misleading.

And some of us who have a sensitivity to lactose may decide against taking lactase supplements. We may instead opt for going along with the wisdom of our bodies, avoiding dairy in all of its common forms, and get our calcium from other sources.

For the normally dairy-sensitive individual, here is a basic group of some other excellent alternative calcium sources:

Figure 26: ALTERNATIVE CALCIUM SOURCES

ALTERNATIVE CALCIUM SOURCES
Bone Broth – see Strong Bones Recipes
Canned fish (sardines, salmon, mackerel) with bones – the bones have the most calcium. Sardines are the smaller fish.
Green leafy vegetables (Bok choy, broccoli, collard & turnip greens, kale, Swiss chard, turnip greens, green beans, etc.
Soybeans, tofu, tempeh, soy yogurt
Yogurt or kefir dairy products – because they are fermented, they might work for some of us (but beware, most these have lots of added sugar)

The MyPlate guidelines suggest that we replace full-fatted dairy products with reduced-fat or fat-free dairy products. One reason is because the fats in dairy products are saturated fats. Dairy products like cream cheese are mainly just fat and don't even count toward our daily recommended servings from the dairy group. There are many other replacements for dairy milk, like almond, cashew, coconut, and soy "milks" we can use to replace dairy milk, but they may not contain much, if any, calcium.

Besides, calcium is really the main nutrient we are looking for in our recommended dairy consumption. How much calcium do we really need, and how else can we get enough of it?

CALCIUM

The Recommended Daily Allowance (RDA) of calcium is 1000 mg. /day for men and 1200 mg. /day for women. But dairy is actually a poor source of ABSORBABLE calcium. Our bodies only absorb about 300-400 mg of the 1000 mg to 1200 mg of the calcium that we may consume from dairy sources.

Excess calcium that is not absorbable by our teeth and bones may be laid down in our arteries. It can also be placed in deposits in other parts of our bodies showing up as funny "lumps" most noticeable just under the skin on arms, legs, or other places. That lump under your skin that you show your doctor and she says "it's just a calcium deposit," that's one place your body puts some of the unusable calcium you eat. This keeps it somewhat locked up and put away in a relatively safe place.

Our bodies also need soluble fats like vitamin D (vitamin D is actually a hormone) for the absorption of our dietary calcium. We can get vitamin D from the sun and from other sources. We'll cover vitamin D in more detail when we look at some Strong Bones Recipes.

For the majority of us who do not tolerate dairy well, we'll also look at some other ingredients we will want to be sure to include that help maximize our calcium absorption, and strengthen our bones.

The concept of a "food-chain" is another issue that appears directly linked to our absorption of calcium from the dairy family. Modernization of farming practices has really shortchanged us in terms of nutrition here. That's because when cows are fed a diet of grains (as is the common practice), their milk lacks many vitamins (like vitamin K) and minerals needed for digestion by humans.

But when cows eat quickly growing young grasses (the way nature intended), the important vitamins and minerals they consume as part of their grass eating diets also become incorporated into their milk. From their milk, we may receive a sufficient supply of the vitamins and minerals our bodies need to better digest that milk in order to use the calcium for our bones and teeth. And if we drink that milk raw, without pasteurization, we may realize health benefits from the Omega 3's that are in that raw milk product.

The young, quickly growing grasses that are the natural food of cows, are loaded with chlorophyll. Chlorophyll is the vital life force of all plants. Chlorophyll is full of vitamin K, essential for the correct use of calcium, among other things. When the calcium we consume is from dairy products that are lacking in vitamin K, the majority of the calcium is not in a usable form and tends to clog our arteries and create those calcium deposits we talked about earlier. But the effects of vitamin K are not limited in scope to just their support of the ways our bodies use calcium.

Vitamin K is also necessary for blood clotting. For instance, frequent nose-bleeds may alert you to low vitamin K levels. Individuals taking warfarin may experience difficulties because that drug interferes with the absorption of vitamin K. "Vitamin K deficiency is manifest as a tendency to bleed excessively. Indeed, many commercially-available rodent poisons [like d-CON®, even with its' "Good Housekeeping" seal of approval] are compounds that interfere with vitamin K and kill by inducing lethal hemorrhage."[92] So you need to also know this: The food chain can be perilous because a dog or cat who eats a rodent who ate the bait laced with the poison, my also die due to bleeding disease caused by the poison that was eaten by that rodent.

But back to our discussion on calcium. We can thank <u>Weston A. Price</u>[93] who spent many years studying, researching, and reporting in great detail about his findings on vitamin K and calcium absorption. More recent scientific research confirms his reports, and may take his research even further.

The journal *Open Heart* published research in October, 2015 by James DiNicolantonio showing that the impact vitamin K has goes even further than the strength of our healthy bones. Dr. DiNicolantonio also credits vitamin K with the "prevention and treatment of arterial calcifications, coronary heart disease and cancer, [as well as] improvements in bone strength and reduced risks of fractures as well as improvements in insulin sensitivity."[94]

So vitamin K does a lot more than keep our strong bones. Vitamin K also can keep our arteries clear as well as provide protection against cancer and heart disease. Not only that, it can improve our insulin sensitivity. This makes assuring an adequate intake of vitamin K an important preventive, as well as a potential alternative healing measure for anyone experiencing insulin resistance, prediabetes, or type 2 diabetes.

But back to Dr. Price. As a dentist doing research, Dr. Price also noticed that the folks in older civilizations did not get as many dental carries as those folks in our current-day societies. And he also noticed, most importantly, that their cows ate foods that just naturally grew in fields, like the tender shoots of young grasses loaded with chlorophylll, the basis of vitamin K.

Some excellent dietary sources of vitamin K include parsley, kale, spinach, Swiss chard, collards, and mustard greens. These can be eaten raw or cooked.

Another thing Weston A. Price noticed about these older civilizations is that they usually consumed the whole animals that they killed for their food. Of course, the bones of these animals were too difficult for humans to chew, but they could make a delicious and highly nutritious soup.

STRONG BONES RECIPES

BONE BROTH

Bone Broth, when prepared from grass-fed animal bones and organic vegetables delivers a much superior form of calcium. Bone Broth can be especially helpful to those with a dairy intolerance. When we enjoy Bone Broth, we even consume the collagen, glucosamine and chondroitin that many purchase as expensive nutritional supplements.

Bone Broth even brings you magnesium, phosphorous, silica, Sulphur, and the trace minerals your body needs to absorb the calcium in your diet.

This makes Bone broth an exceptional source of calcium – and you can easily make it from your kitchen scraps! Save all of your vegetable scraps in the freezer – any trimmings you may have, including things like onion skins. Save the bones from any meats and poultry you have cooked, too. Grass-fed or free-range sourced organic meats and poultry that have been treated to field grazing and not treated with antibiotics or hormones are best.

When you have collected a generous amount of these scraps, place your bones and vegetable scraps into a pot and cover them all with water. Add a tablespoon or two of vinegar to speed the leaching process of getting the minerals out of the bones. Add a bay leaf and a little black pepper. Simmer for 24-36 hours. Why not recycle these would-be wastes into tasty ingredients for better health?

{*Note: If you use an electric crock pot for this, be sure your device does not shut off after 12 hours, as you'll want to simmer this recipe for at least 24 hours. That way all of the goodness will seep out of the bones and into your delicious broth.} *~ End of note.

There is more we can do to maintain our strong bones. Let's look at some other key ingredients, like the minerals we want to be sure to include in our recipes for strong bones.

BORON

Getting enough of the trace mineral boron in your diet is important. Boron is found in fruits, nuts, and vegetables. Some good sources of boron are apples, broccoli and other vegetables, almonds, chickpeas, and avocados. You only need about 2 mg of boron a day. Boron reduces the amount of calcium you lose in your urine, and it also increases the amount of estradiol (the most bioactive form of estrogen). This may be especially important for women.

Keeping fit also helps our bones remain strong. Another bonus to keeping fit is that it also helps manage any symptoms of anxiety or depression we might experience. Depression, heart disease, and adult onset diabetes (type 2 diabetes) are all strongly related. And clinical Depression in women is directly associated with decreased bone mineral density.

Most of us are aware of the adverse effects of smoking and alcohol on our health. The combination of smoking and alcohol consumption (two or more drinks a day) is the worst combination of all. This combination leads to the highest risk for bone mineral loss. Alcohol is very acidic, much like the vinegar we add to the water in our bone broth to leach the minerals out of the bones and into our broth.

PHOSPHOROUS

Our bodies also need phosphorous for our bones and for our healthy teeth. But too much phosphate interferes with the absorption of calcium. The appropriate ratio of calcium to phosphorous in our diets is 2.5:1. That means that we need two and one half times as much calcium as we do phosphorous for our bodies to properly absorb the calcium in our diets.

Nuts, grains, egg yolks, seeds, fish, pork, beef, and beans all contain lots of phosphorous.

It's much more common to have too much phosphorous circulating in our bodies than too little. Folks with weak kidneys may especially have a need to lower their phosphate levels. Eliminating carbonated beverages such as cola is one way to cut down on unnecessary phosphorous in our diet.

Oils are phosphate free. Strawberries, apricots, papaya, cucumber, onion, Romaine and iceberg lettuce are low in phosphorous.

MAGNESIUM

Magnesium is another mineral that our bodies need in order to utilize the calcium in our diets. The appropriate ratio of calcium to magnesium in our diet is 2:1. That means we need twice as much calcium as we do magnesium in order to properly use the calcium in our diets. Some excellent sources of magnesium are avocado, bananas, black beans, broccoli, Brussels sprouts, cooked spinach, dark chocolate, nuts, Swiss chard, unrefined whole grains, yogurt or kefir.

Magnesium is one of those minerals that are truly essential to our lives, so we simply cannot live without it. According to research published in the British Medical Journal *Openheart* in January 2018, titled "Subclinical magnesium deficiency: a principal driver of cardiovascular disease and a public health crisis," our ancestors consumed about 600 mg. of magnesium a day.[95]

But today our average consumption of magnesium is only about 270 mg. a day for a 150lb. person. The USRDA for magnesium is only 310-420 mg. – and for many of us, this may just not be enough. Most of our dietary magnesium comes from the green leafy vegetables we eat. And diets high in protein, calcium and vitamin D increase our need for magnesium. How do you know if you are getting enough magnesium?

Symptoms of magnesium deficiency include: Anxiety, irritability, depression, nervousness, fatigue, inflammation, muscle pain, migraine headache, constipation, insomnia, high blood pressure, type 2 diabetes, undesirable muscle contractions or cramps, weakened bones/osteoporosis and even changes in personality.

While our diets are a good source of magnesium, some people are at risk of magnesium deficiency because of other causes. Gastrointestinal problems may interfere with magnesium absorption, as does alcohol dependence. Those with T2D and the elderly are also at risk. And of course if you aren't getting enough magnesium in your diet as it is, that'll put you at risk as well.

"Magnesium deficiency has been found in 84% of postmenopausal women with osteoporosis diagnosed by low magnesium trabecular bone content and Thoren's magnesium load."[96] That's according to the 2018 study published in the BMJ *Openheart*. But what could be causing all of this osteoporosis?

"Aluminum in the diet may reduce the absorption of magnesium by approximately fivefold, reducing magnesium retention by 41% and causing a reduction of magnesium in the bone."[97] That's how modern researchers describe the results of the research report titled "Effects of dietary aluminum and phosphorus on magnesium metabolism in dairy calves" published in the journal of *Animal Science* in 1990. This research included four groups of animal subjects assigned to four differing diets based on the amounts of magnesium and phosphorous in their feed.

These researchers also tinkered with the amount of phosphorous in the diets of these dairy calves. The study lasted for only 7 weeks. That's all it took to get these measured results. It's important to note that the loss of magnesium was not detected in serum magnesium levels, but *in the bones* of these animals. The bottom line from the researchers is that, "The data indicate that supplemental Al [aluminum] may adversely affect Mg [magnesium] metabolism in calves."[98]

If you give credit to animal studies, then you will seek to remove aluminum contamination. Here are some things you may like to be rid of in order to protect your own magnesium metabolism:

- Aluminum foil used for cooking, storing, or wrapping food
- Bakery products prepared by your grocer or others, as well as those in packages; processed flours, sugar, fats, and any refined foods
- Baking powder (unless the label says aluminum-free)
- Deodorants (read the labels, and look for "aluminum free")
- Other aluminum kitchenware including cookie sheets, cooling racks, baking pans, serving items (read the labels to get aluminum free)
- Prescription and over-the-counter drugs (ask for aluminum-free varieties)
- Teflon pans with an aluminum base

To save some money while you are in the process of switching over to stainless steel, ceramic, glass, or cast iron cookware, parchment paper can be used to line many items of kitchenware to offer some protection. Parchment paper is safe for oven baking.

While the bad news is that our bodies can absorb aluminum through our skin, the good news is that our bodies can also absorb magnesium through our skin, too. Many individuals with those undesirable muscle contractions known as "Restless Leg Syndrome" report dramatic improvement after soaking in an Epsom Salt bath for 30 minutes in the evening before going to bed. (Dissolve 1-2 cupsful into a warm bath as you begin to fill the tub with water.)

Epsom salt (magnesium sulfate) also provides a very inexpensive way to help assure an adequate daily intake of magnesium. A tsp. (or about 5 g.) of Epsom salts dissolved in a glass of water provides about 500 mg. of magnesium.

HAIR MINERAL ANALYSIS

While our bodies can synthesize some vitamins given the right ingredients, our bodies cannot create minerals. The matrix of our bones is 97% protein, but digestive issues may inhibit our ability to absorb the protein our bodies need.

Minerals can be more important than vitamins because they cannot be manufactured by the body. According to Ron Nicklaw, these "minerals are the spark plugs in the chemistry of life. Without optimum mineral levels in the body, the other nutrients are not effectively utilized."[99] If you are interested in preventive strategies, you might consider the benefits of having a hair mineral analysis. Fern's Nutrition offers this specialized personal service, which includes consultation. You can go to www.fernsvitamins.com and click on their hair mineral analysis link for further details. For additional contact information, please see Endnotes.

VITAMIN D

The USRDA for Vitamin D is 400 IU a day for both adults and children. When we are exposed to ultraviolet light (like sunshine), our bodies manufacture vitamin D in our skin. Just ten minutes a day may be all it takes to assure our requirements.

Cod liver oil is the best dietary source of Vitamin D. A tablespoon of cod liver oil contains 1360 IU. Just a teaspoon a day gives you 453 IU of vitamin D at a modest price. As with all oils, be sure to keep it away from heat and light, and preferably in the refrigerator.

Other good sources are fish such as salmon, halibut, carp, and whitefish. Mushrooms are also a good source of vitamin D. Take your fat-soluble vitamins D, A, E, and K with a meal containing fat to help your body transport and absorb their goodness.

OSTEOPOROSIS AND WOMEN'S HEALTH

According the Center for Disease Control, twenty-four and a half percent of women over age 65 have osteoporosis of the femur (upper leg bone) or spine. That's not so bad considering the sedentary lifestyles that have become common in recent decades. Our bones become stronger the more often we put weight on them. That means that sitting at a desk all day is one good way to weaken our bones. So just get up and walk around every fifteen minutes or so, not matter what.

Osteoporosis affects over ten million Americans. Low bone density affects another thirty-four million, leaving them at increased risk for osteoporosis. Osteoporosis fractures usually occur in the hip, spine, or wrist.

The fact is that women are four times more likely to suffer from osteoporosis than men. Out of every ten people with osteoporosis, eight of them are women. That means that eighty percent of those with osteoporosis are women. Osteoporosis might be seen as a natural progression during our aging process, but it sure doesn't have to be.

There are some things we can do that offer preventive advantages. We're going to look at the natural aging process of women and then we'll go on to look at things that both men and women can do to maintain strong bones for a strong and healthy lifestyle in our later years.

MENOPAUSE

Estrogen deficiency is one of the main causes of the loss of bone mass in women during and after menopause. Here is a preventive recommendation for women: Getting a laboratory to give you a copy of your "base line hormone profile" before menopause begins will show you the normal levels of your hormones before their eventual slow decline begins. This is especially important for a woman facing a "surgical menopause." Surgical menopause includes the removal of ovaries, the organs that provide much of the hormones females normally have, like estrogen and testosterone. A base-line hormone profile can offer insight about how much of each hormone you might like to include in hormone replacement therapy (HRT) at a later time in your life – if you decide you'd would like to supplement declining levels. This decline may be natural or surgically induced.

HRT is available in two basic forms, bio-identical, and synthetic. We'll take a look at both of these options now.

SYNTHETIC HORMONES

Synthetic hormones, such as Premarin, which is derived from the urine of pregnant mares, increase the risk of cancer. The Women's Health Initiative study (in 2002) revealed that the synthetic hormone replacements, like Premarin and Prempro increase the risk of breast cancer, stroke, and other problems. Some women using these equine urine based products also report nausea and other digestive disturbances.

A "patch" type of hormone delivery system may be prescribed to relieve your digestive symptoms, but that may offer its' own set of problems, such as a rash from the patch adhesive or other skin irritation. But there is also help available that is more natural. These are called bio-identical hormones.

BIOIDENTICAL HORMONES

Bioidentical hormones are plant based hormones. These are found to be chemically identical to human hormones. But the FDA is at a loss to determine the safety of bioidentical hormones. That's because these *naturally occurring compounds* cannot be patented by drug companies.

When a "drug" cannot be patented, pharmaceutical companies face a major cash loss situation if they develop products containing them and fund the testing of these products. Testing is required for FDA approval. That's why bio-identical hormone replacement products are not tested for safety. But they are effective and without many of the common side-effects of synthetic hormones, since they are biologically identical to our own.

Individually custom designed bio-identical hormone products are also available. These are crafted for your own specific needs by a "Compounding" pharmacy and may be delivered through a cream base. The cream is applied to the skin in a set amount each day, delivering the desired amount of bioidentical hormone to be absorbed through the skin.

Commercially prepared options like Menest (for estrogen) and Methyl-testosterone, or Estratest (for testosterone) are bio-identical options in a pill form that are available through most mainstream pharmacies. These are pharmaceutically produced, standardized, plant-based hormone therapies without the digestive disturbances or side effects of the pregnant mare urine based chemical hormone replacements.

Menopause can be a really confusing time of life because of changes in our hormone levels. We may awaken to "night sweats," have "hot flashes" at inopportune times during the day, and wonder how on earth we will ever be the same again. Our own emotions may even frighten us. This seeming chaos may actually just be due to these hormonal changes. There are some aspects of life that are strictly due to being female. Sometimes just a reassuring voice amid the chaos is all that is needed.

If you are looking for help evaluating your HRT options, the book *"Women's Bodies, Women's Wisdom"* by Christaine Northrup, MD lists hormone replacement options [100] on pages 778 through 786 in detail. If you are on the menopause path, I highly recommend this resource.

If you have other concerns regarding menopause, I recommend Dr. Northrup's book *"The Wisdom of Menopause"*[101]. Both of her works are treasured resources packed with case studies, and loaded with details. Dr. Northrups' works offer insight, comfort, and confidence. And she does not hesitate to face controversial practices head on. Now we'll move on to some things that both women and men can do to maintain strong bones for lifelong active lifestyles.

EXERCISES FOR BALANCE AND BONE STRENGTH IN MEN AND WOMEN

A major debilitating problem for aging populations – and rightly so – is a broken hip. The question we ask is, "did she fall and break her hip, or did her hip break, causing her to fall?"

Hip replacement surgery is very popular and a broken hip can be devastating. Such pain and suffering may be needless with a little preparation and some simple strengthening of our bones.

Bones get stronger when they deal with the mild stress of carrying weight. That's why we talk about weight-bearing exercise so much. Resistance training is good for this, as well as simple weight-bearing exercises, like walking. And weight training can be done at any age to strengthen our bones, no matter what shape they are in.

Falls can cause broken bones – especially the bones of the wrist, spine, and hip. Falls are often caused when someone "loses their balance." Balance is something that we can also improve even as we age, with just a bit of practice. There is a simple exercise that we can do – at any age – that can improve our balance.

This simple exercise taken from the animal kingdom is both weight bearing and also helps us improve our balance at any age – and even children may find this a lot of fun.

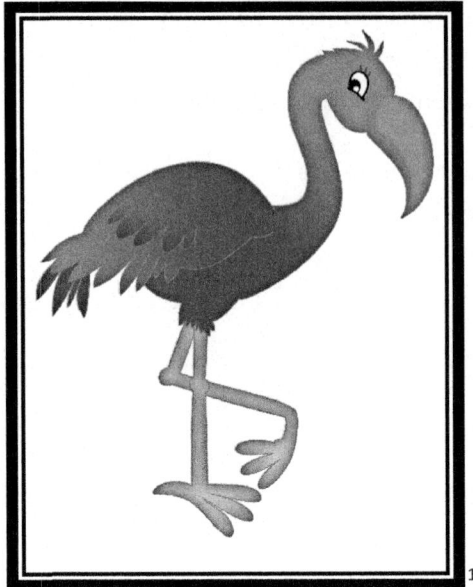

102

Spend just a minute three times a day while balancing on each foot – with your eyes open – to improve your balance. Putting all of your weight on one foot may also increase the bone density in your hips. You can hold on to something (like a walker, counter top, or the back of a chair) to help you gain better balance, as you practice this simple balancing exercise each day. Your body will not only gain better balance, but potentially stronger hips as well.

As with the bio-identical hormone replacement therapy we talked about for women, there is no financial incentive for large-scale testing of this natural and simple exercise. One researcher, Sakamoto, calculated that the effect of standing on one foot for a minute has the same effect on bone density as a 53 minute walk. He further calculated that standing on one foot increases the weight load on the head of the femur (the most frequent site of a break) by a factor of 2.75 over standing on two legs.103

Another simple exercise can be done on a trampoline. Standing in the middle of a mini-tram with your knees bent for just two minutes each day is another great exercise for improving your balance. You can hold on to something for balance if you need to until you get better at balancing on your own.

There is something you will notice while doing either of these simple balancing exercises. All of the muscles in your legs and feet will be getting gentle exercise. You will feel many little muscles being called into play as you maintain your balance. That's because all of these muscles are taking part in balancing your body.

Making these simple exercises habits can go a long way to assuring healthy strong bones. These strong bones will carry you wherever you want to go for all of your active long life.

[1] Yudkin J, Lustig R. 2013. Penguin Books, 36999th Edition. "Pure White and Deadly, How Sugar is Killing Us and What We Can Do to Stop it." https://www.amazon.com/Pure-White-Deadly-Sugar-Killing/dp/0143125184

[2] Seyfried, Thomas, "Cancer as a Metabolic Disease On the Origin, Management, and Prevention of Cancer." June 12, 2012. *John Wiley & Sons*, Hoboken, New Jersey https://www.amazon.com/Cancer-Metabolic-Disease-Management-Prevention/dp/0470584920

[3] United States Department of Agriculture Agricultural Research Service National Nutrient Database for Standard Reference Legacy Release. Accessed at: https://ndb.nal.usda.gov/ndb/search/list
[4] Nutrition data for Corn oil: https://nutritiondata.self.com/facts/fats-and-oils/580/2

[5] Oliveira-de-Lira L, Santos E, Souza R., et al. "Supplementation-Dependent Effects of Vegetable Oils with Varying Fatty Acid Compositions on Anthropometric and Biochemical Parameters in Obese Women." *Nutrients.* 2018 Jul 20;10(7). pii: E932. doi: 10.3390/nu10070932. Accessed 1-12-19 at: https://www.ncbi.nlm.nih.gov/pubmed/30037019

[6] Gillingham L, Harris-Janz S, Jones P. "Dietary monounsaturated fatty acids are protective against metabolic syndrome and cardiovascular disease risk factors." *Lipids.* 2011 Mar;46(3):209-28. doi: 10.1007/s11745-010-3524-y. Epub 2011 Feb 10. Accessed 3-11-19 at: https://www.ncbi.nlm.nih.gov/pubmed/21308420

[7] Zhao J, Lyu C, Gao J, et al. "Dietary fat intake and endometrial cancer risk: A dose response meta-analysis." *Medicine* (Baltimore). 2016 Jul;95(27):e4121. doi: 10.1097/MD.0000000000004121. Accessed 3-11-19 at: https://www.ncbi.nlm.nih.gov/pubmed/27399120

[8] Tan B, Norhaizan M, Liew W. "Nutrients and Oxidative Stress: Friend or Foe?" Oxid Med Cell Longev. 2018; 2018: 9719584. Published online 2018 Jan 31. doi: 10.1155/2018/9719584 PMCID: PMC5831951 PMID: 29643982 Accessed 2-4-19 at: https://www.hindawi.com/journals/omcl/2018/9719584/#B286

[9] United States Department of Agriculture Agricultural Research Service National Nutrient Database for Standard Reference Legacy Release. Accessed at: https://ndb.nal.usda.gov/ndb/search/list

[10] Nutrition data for Corn oil: https://nutritiondata.self.com/facts/fats-and-oils/580/2

[11] https://en.wikipedia.org/wiki/Smoke_point

[12] Ibid.

[13] Institute of Medicine, Food and Nutrition Board. "Dietary reference intakes for energy, carbohydrate, fiber, fat, fatty acids, cholesterol, protein, and amino acids (macronutrients)." *National Academy Press.* Washington, DC: 2005. Accessed 11-23-18 at: https://www.nap.edu/read/10490/chapter/1

[14] Orsavova J, Misurcova L, Ambrozova J. "Fatty Acids Composition of Vegetable Oils and Its Contribution to Dietary Energy Intake and Dependence of Cardiovascular Mortality on Dietary Intake of Fatty Acids." *Int J Mol Sci.* 2015 Jun; 16(6): 12871–12890. Published online 2015 Jun 5. doi: 10.3390/ijms160612871 PMCID: PMC4490476 PMID: 26057750 Accessed on 2-7-19 at: https://www.ncbi.nlm.nih.gov/pmc/articles/PMC4490476/

[15] United States Department of Agriculture Agricultural Research Service National Nutrient Database for Standard Reference Legacy Release. Accessed at: https://ndb.nal.usda.gov/ndb/search/list

[16] Nutrition data for Corn oil: https://nutritiondata.self.com/facts/fats-and-oils/580/2

[17] Simopoulos A. U.S. National Library of Medicine National Institutes of Health *Biomed Pharmacother.* 2002. "The importance of the ratio of omega-6/omega-3 essential fatty acids." Oct;56(8):365-79. Accessed 1-10-19 at: https://www.ncbi.nlm.nih.gov/pubmed/12442909/

[18] Ibid.

[19] United States Department of Agriculture Agricultural Research Service National Nutrient Database for Standard Reference Legacy Release. Accessed at: https://ndb.nal.usda.gov/ndb/search/list

[20] https://www.eatthismuch.com/food/nutrition/corn-oil,300/

[21] Nutrition data for Corn oil: https://nutritiondata.self.com/facts/fats-and-oils/580/2

[22] Kawakami Y, Yamanaka-Okumura H, Naniwa-Kuroki Y, et al. "Flaxseed oil intake reduces serum small dense low-density lipoprotein concentrations in Japanese men: a randomized, double blind, crossover study." *Nutr J.* 2015; 14: 39. Published online 2015 Apr 21. doi: 10.1186/s12937-015-0023-2 PMCID: PMC4409715 PMID: 25896182 Accessed 1-22-19 at: https://www.ncbi.nlm.nih.gov/pmc/articles/PMC4409715/

[23] United States Department of Agriculture Agricultural Research Service National Nutrient Database for Standard Reference Legacy Release. Accessed at: https://ndb.nal.usda.gov/ndb/search/list

[24] Nutrition data for Corn oil: https://nutritiondata.self.com/facts/fats-and-oils/580/2

[25] https://www.eatthismuch.com/food/nutrition/corn-oil,300/

[26] United States Department of Agriculture Agricultural Research Service National Nutrient Database for Standard Reference Legacy Release. Accessed at: https://ndb.nal.usda.gov/ndb/search/list

[27] https://www.eatthismuch.com/food/nutrition/corn-oil,300/

[28] Nutrition data for Corn oil: https://nutritiondata.self.com/facts/fats-and-oils/580/2

[29] U.S. Department of Health & Human Services, National Institutes of Health, Office of Dietary Supplements, "Omega 3 Fatty Acids Fact Sheet for Health Professionals." Updated November 21, 2018. Accessed 12-27-18 at: https://ods.od.nih.gov/factsheets/Omega3FattyAcids-HealthProfessional/#en5

[30] Harris WS. Omega-3 fatty acids. In: Coates PM, Betz JM, Blackman MR, et al., eds. *Encyclopedia of Dietary Supplements*. 2nd ed. London and New York: Informa Healthcare; 2010:577-86.

[31] Cholewski M, Tomczykowa M, Tomczyk M. "A Comprehensive Review of Chemistry, Sources and Bioavailability of Omega-3 Fatty Acids." *Nutrients*. 2018 Nov; 10(11): 1662. Published online 2018 Nov 4. doi: 0.3390/nu10111662 PMCID: PMC6267444 PMID: 30400360. Accessed 2-20-19 at: https://www.mdpi.com/2072-6643/10/11/1662/htm

[32] United States Department of Agriculture Agricultural Research Service National Nutrient Database for Standard Reference Legacy Release. Accessed at: https://ndb.nal.usda.gov/ndb/search/list

[33] Simopoulos A. U.S. National Library of Medicine National Institutes of Health *Biomed Pharmacother*. "The importance of the ratio of omega-6/omega-3 essential fatty acids." 2002 Oct;56(8):365-79. Accessed 12-31-18 at: https://www.ncbi.nlm.nih.gov/pubmed/12442909/

[34] United States Department of Agriculture Agricultural Research Service National Nutrient Database for Standard Reference Legacy Release. Accessed at: https://ndb.nal.usda.gov/ndb/search/list

[35] Nutrition data for corn oil: https://www.eatthismuch.com/food/nutrition/corn-oil,300/

[36] Nutrition data for corn oil: https://nutritiondata.self.com/facts/fats-and-oils/580/2

[37] Chen M, Li Y, Sun Q, et al. U.S. National Library of Medicine, National Institutes of Health. *Am J Clin Nutr.* "Dairy fat and risk of cardiovascular disease in 3 cohorts of US adults."2016 Nov;104(5):1209-1217. Epub 2016 Aug 24. Accessed 1-30-19 at :https://www.ncbi.nlm.nih.gov/pubmed/27557656c

[38] Ibid.

[39] Orsavova J, Misurcova L, Ambrozova J, et al. "Fatty Acids Composition of Vegetable Oils and Its Contribution to Dietary Energy Intake and Dependence of Cardiovascular Mortality on Dietary Intake of Fatty Acids." *Int J Mol Sci.* 2015 Jun; 16(6): 12871–12890. Published online 2015 Jun 5. doi: 10.3390/ijms160612871 Accessed 3-11-19 at: https://www.ncbi.nlm.nih.gov/pmc/articles/PMC4490476/

[40] Finucane O, Lyons C, Murphy A, et al. "Monounsaturated fatty acid-enriched high-fat diets impede adipose NLRP3 inflammasome-mediated IL-1ß secretion and insulin resistance despite obesity." *Diabetes.* 2015 Jun;64(6):2116-28. doi: 10.2337/db14-1098. Epub 2015 Jan 27. Accessed 3-9-19 at: https://www.ncbi.nlm.nih.gov/pubmed/25626736

[41] United States Department of Agriculture Agricultural Research Service National Nutrient Database for Standard Reference Legacy Release. Accessed at: https://ndb.nal.usda.gov/ndb/search/list

[42] Nutrition data for corn oil: https://nutritiondata.self.com/facts/fats-and-oils/580/2

[43] Nutrition data for corn oil: https://www.eatthismuch.com/food/nutrition/corn-oil,300/

[44] Fung J, Moore J. The Complete Guide to Fasting: Heal Your Body Through Intermittent, Alternate-Day, and Extended Fasting. 2016. *Victory Belt Publishing.* https://www.amazon.com/Complete-Guide-Fasting-Intermittent-Alternate-day/dp/1628600012/ref=sr_1_3?keywords=Jason+Fung&qid=1555875425&s=gateway&sr=8-3

[45] Pujol J, Christinat N, Ratinaud Y. "Coordination of GPR40 and Ketogenesis Signaling by Medium Chain Fatty Acids Regulates Beta Cell Function." *Nutrients.* 2018 Apr 12;10(4). pii: E473. doi: 10.3390/nu10040473. Accessed 1-23-19 at: https://www.mdpi.com/2072-6643/10/4/473

[46] Grandl G, Straub L, Rudigier C, et al. "Short-term feeding of a ketogenic diet induces more severe hepatic insulin resistance than an obesogenic high-fat diet." Journal of Physiology. First published: 08 August 2018 https://doi.org/10.1113/JP275173 Accessed 2-20-19 at: https://physoc.onlinelibrary.wiley.com/doi/10.1113/JP275173

[47] Dashti H, Thazhumpal M, Hussein T, et al. "Long-term effects of a ketogenic diet in obese patients." Exp Clin Cardiol. 2004 Fall; 9(3): 200–205. PMCID: PMC2716748 PMID: 19641727 Accessed 2-21-19 at: https://www.ncbi.nlm.nih.gov/pmc/articles/PMC2716748/

[48] Maki K, Hasse W, Dicklin M, et al. "Corn Oil Lowers Plasma Cholesterol Compared with Coconut Oil in Adults with Above-Desirable Levels of Cholesterol in a Randomized Crossover Trial." J Nutr. 2018 Oct 1;148(10):1556-1563. doi: 10.1093/jn/nxy156. Accessed 1-15-19 at: https://academic.oup.com/jn/article/148/10/1556/5094775

[49] Seidelmann F, Claggett B, Cheng S, et al. "Dietary carbohydrate intake and mortality: a prospective cohort study and meta-analysis." The lancet Public Health. Published:August 16, 2018DOI:https://doi.org/10.1016/S2468-2667(18)30135-X Accessed 1-12-19 at: https://www.thelancet.com/journals/lanpub/article/PIIS2468-2667(18)30135-X/fulltext#seccestitle10

[50] Tan B, Norhaizan M, Liew W. "Nutrients and Oxidative Stress: Friend or Foe?" Oxid Med Cell Longev. 2018; 2018: 9719584. Published online 2018 Jan 31. doi: 10.1155/2018/9719584 PMCID: PMC5831951 PMID: 29643982 Accessed 2-4-19 at: https://www.hindawi.com/journals/omcl/2018/9719584/#B286

[51] Ibid.
[52] Sankararaman S, Sferra T. "Are We Going Nuts on Coconut Oil?" Curr Nutr Rep. 2018 Sep; 7(3):107-115. Accessed 1-31-19 at: https://rd.springer.com/article/10.1007/s13668-018-0230-5

[53] Wallace T. "Health Effects of Coconut Oil-A Narrative Review of Current Evidence." Am Coll Nutr. 2018 Nov 5:1-11. doi: 10.1080/07315724.2018.1497562. [Epub ahead of print] Accessed 1-31-19 at: https://www.pubfacts.com/detail/30395784/Health-Effects-of-Coconut-Oil-A-Narrative-Review-of-Current-Evidence

[54] Swanson, R. G., Regents Professor, Department of Food Science, Washington State University, Hexane Extraction in Soyfoods Processing, 2009.

[55] Willett W, Stamper M, Manson J. et al. "Intake of trans fatty acids and risk of coronary heart disease among women." The Lancet VOL 341: MARCH 6, 1993 581-585. Accessed 12-27-18 at: https://pdfs.semanticscholar.org/a766/2837493e4c2aa8ddcf385652b3cb08724bea.pdf

[56] United States Department of Agriculture Agricultural Research Service

National Nutrient Database for Standard Reference Legacy Release. Accessed at: https://ndb.nal.usda.gov/ndb/search/list

[57] Forouhi N, Krauss R, Taubes G, Willett, W. "Dietary fat and cardiometabolic health: evidence, controversies, and consensus for guidance." *BMJ* 2018; 361 doi: https://doi.org/10.1136/bmj.k2139 (Published 13 June 2018) BMJ 2018;361:k2139 Accessed 8-11-18 at: https://www.bmj.com/content/361/bmj.k2139

[58] Dewey C. "Analysis Artificial trans fats, widely linked to heart disease, are officially banned." Washington Post ISSN 0190-8286. 12-21-18. Accessed 12-26-18 at: https://www.washingtonpost.com/news/wonk/wp/2018/06/18/artificial-trans-fats-widely-linked-to-heart-disease-are-officially-banned/?utm_term=.4d26f5b0f1c5

[59] United States Department of Agriculture Agricultural Research Service National Nutrient Database for Standard Reference Legacy Release. Accessed 12-27-18 at: https://ndb.nal.usda.gov/ndb/foods/show/21238?man=&lfacet=&count=&max=25&qlookup=French+fries+&offset=&sort=default&format=Abridged&reportfmt=other&rptfrm=&ndbno=&nutrient1=&nutrient2=&nutrient3=&subset=&totCount=&measureby=&Qv=1.50&Q334409=1&Q334410=1&Q334411=1&Q334412=1.50&Qv=1&Q334409=1&Q334410=1&Q334411=1&Q334412=1.50

[60] The National Academies Press: The National Academies of Sciences Engineering Medicine. Dietary Reference Intakes for Energy Carbohydrate Fiber Fat Fatty acids Cholesterol Protein and Amino acids 2005 Accessed 2-28-19 at: https://www.nap.edu/read/10490/chapter/12#593

[61] US National Library of Medicine; National Center for Biotechnology Information Pub Chem Open Chemistry Database. Accessed 2-28-19 at: https://pubchem.ncbi.nlm.nih.gov/compound/l-isoleucine
[62] Ibid. Accessed 2-29-19 at: https://pubchem.ncbi.nlm.nih.gov/compound/L-leucine
[63] Ibid. Accessed 2-18-19 at: https://pubchem.ncbi.nlm.nih.gov/compound/L-lysine
[64] Ibid. Accessed 2-28-19 at: https://pubchem.ncbi.nlm.nih.gov/compound/L-methionine
[65] Ibid. Accessed 2-28-19 at: https://pubchem.ncbi.nlm.nih.gov/compound/L-phenylalanine
[66] Ibid. Accessed 2-28-19 at : https://pubchem.ncbi.nlm.nih.gov/compound/L-threonine
[67] Ibid. Accessed 2-28-19 at: https://pubchem.ncbi.nlm.nih.gov/compound/L-tryptophan

[68] Ibid. Accessed 3-1-19 at: https://pubchem.ncbi.nlm.nih.gov/compound/L-valine

[69] Ibid. Accessed 3-1-19 at: https://pubchem.ncbi.nlm.nih.gov/compound/L-histidine

[70] Gupta R, Gangoliya S, Singh N. "Reduction of phytic acid and enhancement of bioavailable micronutrients in food grains." J Food Sci Technol. 2015 Feb; 52(2): 676–684. Published online 2013 Apr 24. doi: 10.1007/s13197-013-0978-y PMCID: PMC4325021 PMID: 25694676 Accessed 2-22-19 at: https://www.ncbi.nlm.nih.gov/pmc/articles/PMC4325021/

[71] Basanti C, Kushwaha A, Kumar A. "Sprouting characteristics and associated changes in nutritional composition of cowpea (Vigna unguiculata)." J Food Sci Technol. 2015 Oct; 52(10): 6821–6827. Published online 2015 Apr 14. doi: 10.1007/s13197-015-1832-1 PMCID: PMC4573095 PMID: 26396436 Accessed 2-22-19 at: https://www.ncbi.nlm.nih.gov/pmc/articles/PMC4573095/

[72] United States Department of Agriculture Agricultural Research Service National Nutrient Database for Standard Reference Legacy Release. Accessed at: https://ndb.nal.usda.gov/ndb/search/list

[73] Tan B, Norhaizan M, Liew W. "Nutrients and Oxidative Stress: Friend or Foe?"
Oxid Med Cell Longev. 2018; 2018: 9719584. Published online 2018 Jan 31. doi: 10.1155/2018/9719584 PMCID: PMC5831951 PMID: 29643982 Accessed 2-4-19 at:
https://www.hindawi.com/journals/omcl/2018/9719584/#B286

[74] Ibid.

[75] United States Department of Agriculture Agricultural Research Service National Nutrient Database for Standard Reference Legacy Release. Accessed at: https://ndb.nal.usda.gov/ndb/search/list

[76] Tan B, Norhaizan M, Liew W. "Nutrients and Oxidative Stress: Friend or Foe?" Oxid Med Cell Longev. 2018; 2018: 9719584. Published online 2018 Jan 31. doi: 10.1155/2018/9719584 PMCID: PMC5831951 PMID: 29643982 Accessed 2-4-19 at:
https://www.hindawi.com/journals/omcl/2018/9719584/#B286

[77] United States Department of Agriculture Agricultural Research Service National Nutrient Database for Standard Reference Legacy Release. Accessed at: https://ndb.nal.usda.gov/ndb/search/list

[78] Marventano S, Vetrani C, Vitale M, et al. " Whole Grain Intake and Glycaemic Control in Healthy Subjects: A Systematic Review and Meta-Analysis of Randomized Controlled Trials." Nutrients 2017, 9(7), 769. doi:10.3390/nu9070769 Accessed 7-16-18 at www.mdpi.com/2072-

6643/9/7/769/htm#B62-nutrients-09-00769

[79] Ludwig D, Hu F, Tappy L, Brand-Miller J. "Dietary carbohydrates: role of quality and quantity in chronic disease." *BMJ.*. 2018; 361 doi: ttps://doi.org/10.1136/bmj.k2340 (Published 13 June 2018) Cite this as: BMJ 2018;361:k2340 Accessed 7-23-18 at: https://www.bmj.com/content/361/bmj.k2340

[80] Fuhrman J. *"Fast Food Genocide."* Reprint published Oct. 2017. HarperCollins Publishers. 349 Pgs. https://www.amazon.com/Fast-Food-Genocide-Processed-Killing/dp/0062571214

[81] Hari V. *"The Food Babe Way."* February 10, 2015. Little, Brown and Company. 367 Pgs. https://www.amazon.com/Food-Babe-Way-Younger-Healthy/dp/0316376485

[82] United States Department of Agriculture Agricultural Research Service National Nutrient Database for Standard Reference Legacy Release. Accessed at: https://ndb.nal.usda.gov/ndb/search/list

[83] Wedick N, Pan A, Cassidy A, Rimm E, et al. "Dietary flavonoid intakes and risk of type 2 diabetes in US men and women." *Am J Clin Nutr* 95:925–933, 2012 Accessed 8-15-18 at: https://academic.oup.com/ajcn/article/95/4/925/4576841

[84] Ley S, Schultz M, Hivert M. et. at. Chapter 13: "Risk Factors for Type 2 Diabetes." U.S. Department of Health and Human Services National Institute of Diabetes and Digestive and Kidney Diseases. Accessed on 8-15-18 at: https://www.niddk.nih.gov/about-niddk/strategic-plans-reports/diabetes-in-america-3rd-edition

[85] United States Department of Agriculture Agricultural Research Service National Nutrient Database for Standard Reference Legacy Release. Accessed at: https://ndb.nal.usda.gov/ndb/search/list

[86] Ibid.
[87] Ibid.
[88] Ibid.
[89] Ibid.
[90] Ibid.

[91] Weise E. *USA Today.* "Sixty Percent of Adults Can't Digest Milk." Accessed 8-18-18 at: https://abcnews.go.com/Health/WellnessNews/story?id=8450036

[92] "Vitamin K." Vivo.colostate.edu. 2 Jul 1999 Accessed 1-5-19 at: http://www.vivo.colostate.edu/hbooks/pathphys/topics/vitamink.html

[93] Masterjohn, C. *The Weston A. Price Foundation*. Published Feb. 14, 2018 Accessed 7-23-18 at: https://www.westonaprice.org/health-topics/abcs-of-nutrition/on-the-trail-of-the-elusive-x-factor-a-sixty-two-year-old-mystery-finally-solved/

[94] DiNicolantonio J, Bhutani J, O'Keefe J. "The health benefits of vitamin K" *Open Heart*. 2015; 2(1): e000300. Published online 2015 Oct 6. doi: 10.1136/openhrt-2015-000300 PMCID: PMC4600246 PMID: 26468402 Accessed 1-4-18 at: https://www.ncbi.nlm.nih.gov/pmc/articles/PMC4600246/
[95] DiNicolantonio J, O'Keefe J, Wilson W. "Subclinical magnesium deficiency: a principal driver of cardiovascular disease and a public health crisis." BMJ Open Heart 2018;5:e000668. doi: 10.1136/openhrt-2017-000668 Online issue publication January 13, 2018 Accessed 2-23-19 at: https://openheart.bmj.com/content/5/1/e000668.info
[96] DiNicolantonio J, O'Keefe J, Wilson W. "Subclinical magnesium deficiency: a principal driver of cardiovascular disease and a public health crisis." BMJ Open Heart 2018;5:e000668. doi: 10.1136/openhrt-2017-000668 Online issue publication January 13, 2018 Accessed 2-23-19 at: https://openheart.bmj.com/content/5/1/e000668.info
[97] Ibid.

[98] Neathery M, Crowe N, Miller W, et. Al. *J Anim Sci.* 1990 Apr;68(4):1133-8. Effects of dietary aluminum and phosphorus on magnesium metabolism in dairy calves. Accessed 3-4-19 at: https://www.ncbi.nlm.nih.gov/pubmed/2332387?dopt=Abstract

[99] Ron Nicklaw, CNC. Fern's Nutrition. 2019. 16932 Gothard, Suite H Huntington Beach, CA. 92647 (714) 841-5349 For hair mineral analysis: https://www.fernsvitamins.com/vitamins/Home/hair_analysis.html

[100] Northrup, C. "Women's Bodies, Women's Wisdom Creating Physical and Emotional Health and Healing" *Bantam Books*. 1998:777-786.
[101] Northrup C. "The Wisdom of Menopause, Creating Physical and Emotional Health during the Change". *Hay House, Inc.*: Revised Updated Edition. January 3, 2012.

[102] https://openclipart.org/image/800px/svg_to_png/227691/1442549721.png
[103] Sakamoto K. Effects of unipedal standing balance exercise on the prevention of falls and hip fracture. *Clin Calcium*. 2006 Dec;16(12):2027-32. Accessed 7-26-18 at: https://www.ncbi.nlm.nih.gov/pubmed/17142934

NUTRIENT ESSENTIALS

A

Acidosis, 49

Adenosine triphosphate (ATP), about, 64

Aging, 16
  diets for longevity, 53
  health and, 89
  osteoporosis and, 130
  strong bones and, 132

Alcohol dependence
  magnesium deficiency and, 126

Algae, Algal oil, 35

Allergies, 55, 89

Almonds, 14, 89, 124

Aluminum
  about, 126
  contamination, removal steps, 127
  magnesium metabolism and, 126, 128

Alzheimer's disease, 54

American College of Nutrition, The, 54

Amino acids,calculating daily needs, 62

Animal Science, Journal, 127

Animal-based diets, guidance, 53

Anthocyanin, dietary sources of, 90

Antioxidants, 2, 16, 82, 89
  free radicals and, 89
  oxidative stress and, 74, 89

Anxiety
  magnesium and, 126

Apples, 89, 90, 124

Apricots, 125

Arachidonic Acid, 19

Are You Sweet Enough Already?
  (Lickus), 75

Artificial Intelligence, 54
  genetic variances and, 54

Astaxanthin
  benefits of, 36

how to buy, 36

Asthma, 39

Auditory function, 53

Autoimmune diseases, 18
  and Omega 6/
    3 Ratios, 24

Autophagy,about, 88

Avocados, 14, 124, 125

B

Bald patches, 54

Better Butter Recipe, 14

Bioflavonoids, about, 89

Bio-identical hormones
  about, 131

Biomarkers, 26

Biomed Pharmacotherapy, Journal, 24

*Biomedicine and Pharmacotherapy,
  Journal of*, 38

Biotin (B7), deficiency symptoms, 80

Blood clotting
  important nutrients for, 22

Blood sugar levels
  insulin and, 87

Blueberries, 90

Bone loss, 54

Boron, daily needs, 124

Brain function, important nutrients for, 23

Bran, about, 78

British Medical Journal, The, 58, 78, 125

Broccoli, 124

C

Calcium
  absorption, increasing, 121
  bone broth and, 123

P

OUNCE TO GRAM CONVERSIONS

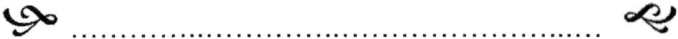

OUNCES	GRAMS (Rounded)
.33	9
.5	14
.99	28
1	28
1.34	38
1.5	43
1.76	50
2.12	60
2.82	80
4.23	120
5.29	150

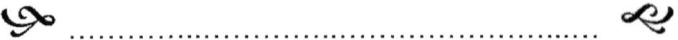

OTHER BOOKS BY THIS AUTHOR

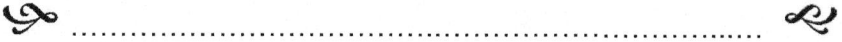

Cheat Sheet Simply for USA Foods

Cheat Sheet Simply for Canadian Foods

Cheat Sheet Simply for UK Foods

Low Glycemic Happiness: 120 Recipes for Blood Sugar Control

Are You Sweet Enough Already? Ten Dessert Recipes for Blood Sugar Control

Beyond the Knife: Alternatives to Surgery

NUTRIENT ESSENTIALS

NOTES

Printed in Dunstable, United Kingdom

70229479R00097